A Child's Journey to Recovery

Delivering Recovery

Series edited by Patrick Tomlinson, Strategic Development Director, SACCS

This is an essential series on practice for all professionals and parents involved in providing recovery for traumatized children and young people. Each book offers a practical and insightful introduction to an aspect of SACCS' unique and integrated approach to children traumatized by sexual, physical and emotional abuse.

also in the series

The Child's Own Story
Life Story Work with Traumatized Children
Richard Rose and Terry Philpot
Foreword by Mary Walsh, co-founder and Chief Executive of SACCS
ISBN 978 1 84310 287 8

Reaching the Vulnerable Child
Therapy with Traumatized Children
Janie Rymaszewska and Terry Philpot
Foreword by Mary Walsh, co-founder and Chief Executive of SACCS
ISBN 978 1 84310 329 5

Living Alongside a Child's Recovery
Therapeutic Parenting with Traumatized Children
Billy Pughe and Terry Philpot
Foreword by Mary Walsh, co-founder and Chief Executive of SACCS
ISBN 978 1 84310 328 8

also by Patrick Tomlinson

Therapeutic Approaches in Work with Traumatised Children and Young People
Theory and Practice
Patrick Tomlinson
Foreword by Paul van Heeswyk
ISBN 978 1 84310 187 1

of related interest

Shattered Lives
Children Who Live with Courage and Dignity
Camila Batmanghelidjh
ISBN 978 1 84310 603 6

Fostering Attachments
Supporting Children who are Fostered or Adopted
Kim Golding
ISBN 978 1 84310 614 2

Helping Children to Build Self-Esteem
A Photocopiable Activities Book, Second Edition
Deborah M. Plummer
Illustrated by Alice Harper
ISBN 978 1 84310 488 9

Self-Esteem Games for Children
Deborah Plummer
Illustrated by Jane Serrurier
ISBN 978 1 84310 424 7

Talking with Children and Young People about Death and Dying, Second Edition
Mary Turner
Illustrated by Bob Thomas
ISBN 978 1 84310 441 4

A Child's Journey to Recovery

Assessment and Planning with Traumatized Children

Patrick Tomlinson and Terry Philpot

Foreword by Mary Walsh

Jessica Kingsley Publishers
London and Philadelphia

First published in 2008
by Jessica Kingsley Publishers
116 Pentonville Road
London N1 9JB, UK
and
400 Market Street, Suite 400
Philadelphia, PA 19106, USA

www.jkp.com

Library of Congress Cataloging in Publication Data
Tomlinson, Patrick, 1962-
 A child's journey to recovery : assessment and planning with traumatized children / Patrick Tomlinson
and Terry Philpot ; foreword by Mary Walsh.
 p. ; cm. -- (Delivering recovery series)
 Includes bibliographical references.
 ISBN-13: 978-1-84310-330-1 (pb. : alk. paper) 1. Psychic trauma in children--Diagnosis. 2. Psychic
trauma in children--Treatment. 3. Child mental health services. 4. Psychiatric social work.
 [DNLM: 1. Child Abuse--therapy--Case Reports. 2. Stress Disorders, Traumatic--therapy--Case
Reports. 3. Child. 4. Needs Assessment--Case Reports. 5. Social Work, Psychiatric--methods--Case Reports.
6. Stress Disorders, Traumatic--etiology--Case Reports. WM 172 T659c 2008] I. Philpot, Terry. II. Title. III.
Delivering recovery.
 RJ506.P66T647 2008
 618.92'8521--dc22

                                                                            2007028457

British Library Cataloguing in Publication Data
A CIP catalogue record for this book is available from the British Library

ISBN 978 1 84310 330 1

Printed and bound in Great Britain by
Athenaeum Press, Gateshead, Tyne and Wear

To Georgia for her support and encouragement.

Patrick Tomlinson

To my favourite sisters – Sr Gemma LSA, Sr Anne Mary
LSA and Sr Adele LSA – with fond memories of Worcester
and the summer of '06, and remembering the late
Sr Elizabeth LSA.

Terry Philpot

A Note and Acknowledgements

The names of the children and young people mentioned in this book have been changed, along with any details which might identify them.

As with the three previous books in this series, for ease of reading we have referred to a child and young person as 'she' and all adults as 'he', except where, in the case of mother or other female adult, it has been necessary to be specific.

We would like to thank Mary Walsh, chief executive, SACCS, for her support for this series; Janie Rymaszewska, Richard Rose, Ann Pugh, John Baker, Billy Pughe, Barbara Jones, Kimberley Newton and Carolyn Kartal, all of whom have been involved in the development and management of the SACCS Recovery Assessment and Plan; Lorraine Easterbrook for the use we have made of her work analysing assessment methods, which we gratefully acknowledge.

We should also like to express our thanks to Jessica Kingsley, managing director, Jessica Kingsley Publishers, and Steve Jones, commissioning editor, for help and advice.

Contents

Foreword

For the past 20 years SACCS has been developing a programme to work therapeutically with children who have been traumatized through abuse and neglect. In the beginning this was pioneering work in a context where sexual abuse was a relatively new phenomenon. We saw children who might have been abused and conducted assessments for local authorities and for the courts. These assessments were based on the best possible information about the child's history and knowledge of her experience and distress; the level of emotional development; and, through innovative techniques especially developed to communicate with children, a thorough understanding of the child's needs and her wishes and feelings.

Since those early days we have developed a range of services to help this very vulnerable group of children to recover from their emotional injuries. In the same way as a child with a physical injury needs treatment if she is going to recover, so it is with children who have sustained emotional injuries, usually at the hands of one or both parents, through no fault of their own. And just as a physical injury, if left, will heal, albeit in a distorted way, so will emotional injuries, but the distortions that the child will be left with will not be a limp or a weak limb, but rather distortions in the way that they think and feel. These distortions may have long and wide-reaching effects, and may determine the course of the child's life, and the life of others whom that child may come into contact with. It may mean that she becomes aggressive, withdrawn, highly unpredictable in her behaviour and difficult to manage. She may be self-destructive and suicidal. She may run away, or destroy everything that is important to her. She may pose a sexual risk to others, both now and in the future. She may be driven by abject terror, unable to trust others and living in a constant state of inner chaos. These are children living at the margins, and because of their behaviour, which some see as challenging, they are identified not as victims, which is what they are, but rather as the problem itself.

Whatever the nature of the injury, it is crucial that it is identified correctly and based on the best possible information at the assessment stage, and that decisions and plans made for the child's recovery are based on that information. The assessment and recovery plans need to be reviewed at regular intervals to ensure that the hypothesis was correct and that the child is now on the road to recovery.

Patrick Tomlinson and I have spent the last five years writing the SACCS' recovery programme, with the help of many others within the company. This is a manual on how to deliver recovery to children who have been traumatized by abuse early in their lives. The programme identifies 24 outcomes for recovery, which may be organized into six broad areas to focus on. The SACCS' assessment based on these six areas is routinely carried out on each child, every six months, and is completed by different parts of the recovery team – therapeutic parenting, the therapy and the life-story work. Those responsible for this – the key worker and other staff, the therapist and the life-story worker – work together in an integrated way, holding the child and her potential for healing, and regularly review her progress. From this assessment comes the child's individual recovery plan.

Patrick Tomlinson and Terry Philpot have written a sensitive and comprehensive description of assessment from an historical and eco-logical perspective, and stress the vital importance of getting it right for the child. They have highlighted the consequence of understand-ing the child's history and the impact that that has had on her emotional and physical development, as well as discussing the signifi-cance of joined-up working for the recovery of the child. Furthermore, they have portrayed a model of assessment with illustrations of how it has been applied in practice. My hope would be that this book can become an exemplar of how to use assessment to help children to recover from their emotional injuries.

By putting the child at the centre of everything that we do, and defining outcomes so that we can recognize what a recovering child might look like, in order that she may maximize her potential, it is then possible to assess and plan appropriately, and make decisions, sometimes brave ones, to meet these outcomes.

The only reason we are in this work is to help children to achieve positive outcomes and take their place in society. In order to do this effectively we must have a clearly defined methodology, underpinned by theory, informed by the child and based on a good assessment, strong decision making, planning and an integrated approach.

Mary Walsh
Co-founder and Chief Executive of SACCS

Introduction

According to Easterbrook (2006), 'Assessment appears to be important not only in the gathering of information but in making sense of it' (p.39). If this book achieves nothing else, our hope will be that we will demonstrate not only the truth but the importance of that statement. For assessment is something that is frequently misunderstood, a failing which is then compounded by how it is conducted. Another aim of this book, then, is to show that how a child should be assessed and who is responsible for this are key to successful assessment.

This is not a book which intends to be prescriptive but offers examples of good practice and up-to-date thinking on its subject, and explains the context in which assessment takes place: who the children are and how they function; organizational considerations; and the history of assessment. It will offer a link between theory and practice. This is particularly important as we are mindful that 27 years ago Rowe (1980) warned against developing practice in a theoretical vacuum. Writing of fostering, she said that it lacked a theoretical underpinning and that 'practice wisdom' would not suffice if services were to be integrated and professional. The other side of that coin is another aspect of this book that we wish to stress: its reliance on evidence. This is in keeping with the now well-established emphasis on evidence-based practice.

We will make explicit the causal links between assessment of need, the implementation of plans to meet the identified need and the outcomes for traumatized children who receive a specialized therapeutic service. We hope to show, too, that assessment is not finite, one-off or static; it is not just an act that leads to a next step (other than, of course, in the sense of identifying a service which the child requires). Assessment is a continuing process that allows us to evaluate how successful the initial assessment was, how effective is the treatment offered and what modifications, if any, are then required. But the value of assessment does not even end with the child for whom it was intended because it can teach us about future work and interventions. Cox and Bentovim (2000) even go as so far as to call it 'therapeutic' and, in the case of work with families, say, 'It should enable those involved to gain fresh perspectives on their family situation, which are in themselves therapeutic'.

The only justification for an assessment process is that it should lead to positive outcomes. It is important to understand what we mean by outcomes and where they stand in the whole paraphernalia of other measures like inputs and modern management techniques, such as performance indicators. This is because it is very important not only that the focus is on an individual child but that it is on precisely what is meant to be achieved with her, how that achievement is measured and that we are not distracted by confusion about terminology and method.

Rather than provide, as with other books in this series, a series of case examples (although case references are made from time to time), we have written an appendix which shows the progress of one child, whom we have called Grace. We write in some detail of her family background and influences revealed by the life-story work. We then go on to show, also in some detail, the process and outcomes from three assessments, in the context of assessment generally. This shows not only in words how assessment can work and what it can produce but also the use of the visualization of Grace's progress through the spider diagram, a tool described in Chapter 5.

Along with Easterbrook's point about seeing assessment as something which helps us to understand, one of our central tenets is that assessment for the children about whom we write is not a role for an individual alone. It is a group or a team task, which, by drawing together different perspectives from different disciplines, enables the creation of a holistic understanding of the child, of the child as a person who is more than the sum of her problems and achievements. This requires an integrated approach which we will discuss.

Although this book is about children and, most specifically, about children traumatized through physical, emotional and sexual abuse and neglect, our belief is that the assessment and planning processes described can be adapted and applied in different settings, not only with other groups of children but also with adults.

Creating services tailored to meet the needs of individuals who use them has been an aspiration of policy documents, reports, White Papers and government pronouncements for 20 or more years. The persistence of public service reform, the continuing revolution which governments have promoted for about the same length of time, shows that this aspiration remains far from realization. And yet there is no alternative. We might as well not have services if they do not meet the needs of those who use them because they help no one, harm some and waste valuable resources. Assessment is not about groups, it is about an individual. Get the assessment right, which means understanding its purpose and how it is to be conducted, and this lays the foundation from which all else can fall into place. As Buckley (2007) has argued, 'The process by which assessment is carried out will determine its capacity to be effective' (p.5).

CHAPTER 1

Assessment
What it is and How it has Developed

Assessment is a common part of everyday life. It is a process by which we make decisions, large and small; a process by which we take action by trying to understand where we are and what our future needs (or those of others) are and how we can reach them by defining and obtaining the resources that are needed to do so.

In the management of organizations, volumes are devoted to ways of understanding where we are, how we got there and what signposts there are to the future. Yet assessment is too often regarded by practitioners as something fairly straightforward, almost mechanical – this is the service user's situation, this is what he or she needs and this is the solution in terms of the service to be offered. Such a superficial approach has led to enormous problems across the range of social care services. With regard to the care for children, a failure to understand the facts (which is key to proper and thorough continuing assessment) has led to situations which range from the tragic consequences of children left inappropriately with abusive parents to the damaging instability suffered by children and young people placed in inappropriate care placements that then break down.

One of the pitfalls of assessment in social work has been a tendency to view it as a wholly objective process. This is something which we seek to avoid throughout this book by pointing to both the problems arising from treating it as such and how it *should* be regarded.

This dangerous tendency of seeing assessment as objective has been highlighted by Milner and O'Byrne (2002), when they say:

> gathering information, sifting it carefully and coming to an 'objective' and 'accurate' conclusion is by no means as unproblematic as this suggests; assessment has never been the scientific activity that many writers pretended. (p.8)

Although in the next chapter we look more fully at outcomes, it is relevant at this point to say that Parry and Richardson (1996), in a Department of Health strategic review of policy and psychotherapy services, might have been making a general point about all social care services when they said that therapies could no longer decline to subject themselves to evidence-based research and that practitioners and researchers had to accept the challenge of evidence-based practice, 'one result of which is that treatments which are shown to be ineffective are discontinued' (p.43).

Thus, a concern for outcomes and evidence has become a cornerstone of the modernization of social care with its stress on people-centred and responsive services. This derives from work in the 1980s and early 1990s which emphasized evidence-based practice and measuring incomes. As Aldgate and colleagues (2006) say, 'practice wisdom is a useful, indeed, an essential aid, but it is insufficient unless allied to a firmly based coherent body of knowledge' (pp.56–57).

With such concerns abounding, assessment has to be regarded as essential because it is the foundation for intervention but, in its turn, a concentration on outcomes and evidence has influenced how assessment is carried out. Thus, Ward's (2004) axiom when referring to work with children stands us in good stead in any situation, 'You can have assessment without treatment but you certainly can't have treatment without assessment' (p.9). Ward says that 'assessment for treatment' is:

> the process of making sense of current available experience to help you have some idea of what is going on in your interactions with the child in order to modify, interrupt, emphasize or even ignore certain aspects of the dynamic. (p.9)

But, first, what is assessment? Adcock (2001) defines it as:

> the collection and evaluation of information relevant to an identi-
> fied purpose. Assessment has several phases which overlap and lead
> into planning, action and review:
>
> - the acquisition of information
>
> - exploring facts and feelings
>
> - putting meaning to the situation
>
> - reaching an understanding with the family wherever possible,
>   of what is happening, to include problems, strengths and
>   difficulties and their impact on the child
>
> - drawing up an analysis of the child's needs and the parenting
>   capacity as a basis for formulating a plan. (p.76)

However, as we imply above, it should be pointed out that assessment is
not a neutral concept, and one of the intentions of this book is to show
that there are different ways in which it is conducted, not all of them
conducive to providing the necessary service. Horwath (2001) shows
how assessment and intervention have narrowed with the increasing
concern about child protection. She quotes Stevenson (1998) as stating
that this has led to an 'individualistic model for understanding, and even
for constructing the very problem, rather than an emphasis on external
factors' (p.27).

Before this, though, there had been concern that too often assessment perceived children as the sum of their problems, something wholly
opposed to the 'ecological' assessment whereby the child is seen in
relation to her world, family and circumstances. A 'traditional' approach
to assessment has been found to concentrate on searching for the origins
of past problems (Sinclair, Garrett and Berridge 1995). The corollary of
this, of course, is that this kind of assessment does not seek to identify
the strengths of service users, something that was highlighted by the
Department of Health (DoH) and Department for Education and
Employment (DfEE) (2000) document, *Framework for Assessment of*

Children in Need and Their Families, which encouraged a move from problem-identification to building on the strengths of a family.

Well-being

In seeking positive factors which go to make an assessment, well-being is a comparatively new concept in children's services and one popularized by the Green Paper, *Every Child Matters*, (HM Treasury 2003). It is not something which is applied only to children. Politicians, notably following the lead of the academic Richard Layard (2005), have started to talk generally about concepts of happiness and well-being, and people feeling good about life, which they see (in their rhetoric at least) as being what the goals of government policies should be concerned with. This may be seen perhaps as a response to a widespread, if not always well-articulated feeling that an over-riding regard for material well-being, especially in a consumer and materialistic society that regards image as important, shopping as a pastime and spending as a goal, is unsatisfying, and, indeed, may lead to various personal and social problems.

It is not difficult to see why well-being is a natural component of children's policies; perhaps it is more surprising as to why it has taken so long to be 'discovered'. It is axiomatic in any work with children – from social work to education, therapy to parenting – that the only environment in which children can thrive is one which offers love, comfort, stimulation and challenge. It is one where relationships with carers and teachers as much as neighbours, parents and other family members are important, and where reciprocity is stressed – the Green Paper (HM Treasury 2003) has 'making a contribution' as one of its five outcomes for children. The process of socialization, which has long been a standard of books on parenting as much as the focus of researchers and the concern of clinicians, is one which underpins and is key to well-being.

The integration of children's departments and education departments was based on a belief that it would bring together professionals to offer a holistic service to children and thus enhance their potential and so their well-being. Enjoyment, play, creativity and communication, especially in the early years, are seen as a firm foundation for children, although, it has to be said, that it is not long before children enter formal education and these activities are set aside in favour of acquiring skills and having to sit tests.

Jordan (2007) sees the concern for well-being particularly evident in the shift in the criteria used by inspectors. The new perspective, he says, is one which stems from the emphasis on well-being. Inspectors' reports on day nurseries dwell on whether they 'demonstrate a sense of belonging'; whether children are 'playing well together, co-operatively and negotiating well during their play'. How staff interact with children and respond to their needs is remarked upon (p.142).

Aldgate and colleagues (2006) make the point that in the field of psychology the concept of wellness has been around for a considerable time. It is something which embraces both mental and physical health in children and adolescents. They refer back to Kelly (1974) as providing a good summary of what it means:

> The work of psychologists is moving from an emphasis upon the troubles, the anxieties, the sickness of people, to an interest in how we acquire positive qualities, and how social influences contribute to perceptions of well-being, personal effectiveness, and even joy. There will be signs that, in the future, psychologists less and less will be viewing us as having diseases. Instead, the psychological view will be one of persons in process over time and as participants in social settings. (p.1)

Thus, a child's well-being, her reactions to others, how she relates to them, her sense of belonging, creativity and enjoyment, and her ability to give as well as to receive should form part of an assessment.

The meaning of assessment

When children have suffered harm, assessment gains a special importance because it is a means of avoiding interventions which have proved unsuccessful; at the same time it maintains the child's safety and does all it can to obtain the best outcome (Aldgate *et al.* 2006, p.267). A commitment to the evidence allows practitioners to think more clearly about assessment and what children's needs are and how they can be met.

And so Ward (2004) (rightly) sees assessment not as a one-off initial action but as a tool to take us forwards, one which informs us during treatment and allows us to modify what we do and respond to what is happening to the child who is being treated by, first, taking into account her needs. In the therapeutic process, then, treatment and assessment are partners, they go hand in hand; assessment does not merely guide us to what is the most appropriate treatment and is then left behind, it is a part of the treatment because it is informing what is done by acting as a monitor.

But what we want to emphasize in this book, indeed, something which underpins everything we say about assessment, is that it is not only the practitioner (usually a social worker) who first has contact with the child who needs assessment skills: those are required by everyone who has contact with the child. This is because, first, the model that we will describe is based on a shared or joint assessment and, second, because assessment is the means by which staff in all services for children (not only those in a particular team) are able to judge the success or failure of their actions and interventions. For all of them, too, this assessment must be informed by the views of children themselves. The other important principle is the point made by Dockar-Drysdale (1993), 'I am advocating a therapy based on *needs* rather than *symptoms*' (p.52) (her italics). To do otherwise is to make a basic mistake, which is to see a child in terms of her symptoms rather than as a child, and to regard treating symptoms as more important than meeting needs.

The well-researched, holistic assessment, with its reflective plan, is the antithesis of what Perry and Szalavitz (2006) call 'quick fixes'. These authors explain this by saying:

> Troubled children are in some kind of pain – and pain makes people irritable, anxious and aggressive. Only patient, loving, consistent care works. There are no short-term miracle cures. This is as true for the child of three or four as it is for the teenager. Just because a child is older does not mean a punitive approach is more appropriate or

effective. Unfortunately, again, the system doesn't recognize this. It tends to provide quick fixes, and when those fail then there are long punishments. We need programs and resources that acknowledge that punishment, deprivation, and force merely traumatize children and exacerbate their problems. (p.244)

A holistic or ecological assessment of a child can only come about by a multi-disciplinary and multi-agency assessment. It is not sufficient or helpful, for example, for schools to look only at a child's educational development or social workers to be concerned solely with the family circumstances. Aldgate *et al.* (2006) say, 'nothing can be taken for granted in looking at children's development and an approach to assessment that emphasizes dimensions and intertwining influences from many sources is essential' (p.34).

Strengths and weaknesses of assessment

Ward (2004) says, 'when you look to the literature on assessment, what you tend to find is that it encourages you to think broadly rather than deeply' (p.4). Assessment is a basis for intervention and a means of securing the best outcomes for children. In order to understand where assessment has come from, the possibilities which it offers and how it may be developed it is helpful to look at two assessment methods devised specifically for vulnerable children.[1]

The introduction of the Assessment Framework (Department of Health and Department for Education and Employment 2000) had the primary aim of improving the quality of assessments, made not only by social workers but by all professionals working with children.

In remembering this we should also take account of the context of a wider and earlier history. Assessment is emphasized in a number of major pieces of legislation as a critical process: the Education Reform Act 1988; the Children Act 1989; the NHS and Community Care Act 1990; the Criminal Justice Act 1991; and Education Act 1993 (Milner and O'Byrne 2002). However, what was lacking was an overarching approach, rather than models to suit different groups and situations. That many service users of all ages found themselves in multiple situations and that social workers work within different professional locations were entirely ignored. This is as true for children and young people as for adults. The national assessment framework is discussed below.

But, to step back further in time, Dockar-Drysdale's needs assessment in 1970 was important in that it was the first one of which we are aware that focused specifically on the child's emotional development and how to treat children who had been severely damaged by abuse and deprivation. Dockar-Drysdale also emphasized the importance of the whole team being involved in the assessment process. This is key to this book because, as we have said, we describe an assessment which is arrived at collectively so that the child can be seen holistically.

The other assessment discussed below is the Boxall Profile. This is of interest because it is widely used yet was developed for use in the classroom and was completed by one person (the teacher). This has its disadvantages, but it can also be completed by a team which, we believe, strengthens its use for the purposes we describe.

After considering these two assessments, two others are described: the National Children's Bureau assessment model and the government's Common Assessment Framework.

Dockar-Drysdale's Needs Assessment

The devising of a needs assessment by Dockar-Drysdale in 1970 came after the many years' experience gained as founder and director of the Mulberry Bush School from 1948 to 1963, working with what were then called 'severely disturbed and deprived children' and her later time as consultant psychotherapist to the school (Dockar-Drysdale 1968, 1973). Dockar-Drysdale distinguished the differences between a referral needs assessment and a continuing needs assessment. Her needs assessment sought to classify children on arrival at the school as either 'integrated' or 'unintegrated' (Winnicott 1962). This, and looking at what stage of integration the child had reached, would allow professionals, believed Dockar-Drysdale, to see what her needs were and to work out how they could be met.

Only a group of residential workers who had lived with a child for at least three to four weeks could answer the questions which would determine how the child was to be categorized. A senior worker would lead the group, ask and explain the questions and record the answers. This group assessment was critical to Dockar-Drysdale (1970), who wrote, 'all needs assessments must, in my view, be made by a group, *never* by an individual collecting information or depending upon interview procedure'(p.94).

The two most important questions to decide whether a child was 'integrated' or 'unintegrated' were, first: Does the child panic? That is, has she an 'unthinkable anxiety' which is almost a physical condition? Second: Is the child disruptive – does she break up activities between others? An affirmative answer to these questions meant that the child was 'unintegrated'. There were then four further categories into which the child could be put by asking more questions. These categories were 'frozen', 'archipelago', 'false-self' and 'caretaker-self'.

The first question for the last four categories was: What is the 'syndrome of deprivation'? That is, how did the child express or experience guilt, dependence on others, merger, empathy, stress, communication, identification, depression, aggression. The remaining three questions were about the child's capacity for play, learning and self-preservation.

The answers to these questions were not 'yes' or 'no' but, rather, stemmed from the workers' actual experience of living with, and being close to the child. But from them it would, as Easterbrook (2006) says, be 'usually quite possible to make a good guess at the *stage of integration* [Easterbrook's emphasis] reached' (p.13).

A general list of needs went with each classification and from this was formulated the best way to treat each child. For example, the category for a 'frozen' child would have needs best met by 'containment'. The treatment programme would then detail how the need for containment could be met.

Children who were 'integrated' also had needs that were detailed, but these were considered to be far more individual in nature.

Easterbrook (2006) says:

> the strength of this assessment lies in the fact that the people who
> know how it feels to live with the child are the 'experts' in deter-
> mining into which category a child fits. A senior person is available
> to help as a guide through the assessment but ultimately it is the
> workers who own the classification and can begin to own the
> treatment. There are clear guidelines for how to meet the needs of a
> child once classified and the treatment plan appears to be very
> straightforward. (pp. 13–14)

However, Easterbrook (2006) also points to the assessment's shortcom-
ings, which she finds to be the 'fact that classification leads to a pre-
scribed treatment plan which has been designed by an expert
(Dockar-Drysdale) may leave some workers feeling quite constricted
and unable to use any of their own creativity' (p. 14). Easterbrook also
points out that the needs of the children who are classified as
'unintegrated' appear to be clearer than those classified as 'integrated'.

Boxall Profile

Interestingly, while the Cotswold Community continued to make use of
Dockar-Drysdale's needs assessment, this was no longer so for her old
school, the Mulberry Bush. It has been replaced by the Boxall Profile,
which was originally devised as a structured observational tool to assist
teachers to plan a focused intervention in the classroom.

Marjorie Boxall, an educational psychologist, set up nurture groups
in some schools in socially deprived areas of London to help children
who were showing early signs of emotional and behavioural difficulties.
The idea was to provide a structured and predictable environment in
which the children could begin to trust adults and learn within small
special classes with specially trained staff. According to Bennathan and
Boxall (1998) the profile was developed because 'teachers wanted a
more precise way of assessing need, planning intervention and
measuring progress' (p.4). It was soon being used throughout the whole
school.

The profile received a boost in 1997 when the Department for Education and Employment (DfEE) said that experience showed its usefulness in assisting inclusiveness, enhancing teachers' skills in managing children with emotional and behavioural difficulties, and in developing strategies that lead to effective early intervention.

The profile has three parts: developmental strands, the diagnostic profile and factors likely to affect the scores.

There are 34 descriptions of behaviour in the first two parts, which are scored and entered on the corresponding histogram. Aspects of the developmental process of the early years are described in Section 1 while behaviours that inhibit or interfere with the child's satisfactory involvement in school appear in Section 2. Scoring for each question is between 0 and 4, and each section has a key to scoring.

The developmental strands identify two clusters – organization of experience and internalization of control – each of which has five sub-clusters. (The histogram represents the child's level of functioning visually and each sub-cluster is represented in a column. There is a shaded area which shows a comparative average score for competently functioning children.)

Each of the 34 descriptions is scored to a particular sub-cluster and each group to a cluster. For example, questions 14, 21 and 26 are in the sub-cluster 'Participates constructively'. That sub-cluster, in turn, belongs to the cluster 'Organization of Experience'. The profile offers an interpretation for each sub-cluster of what the score in that particular sub-cluster shows. For these scorings a high score indicates an interested and purposeful involvement with people and events, and some autonomy of functioning and learning.

There are three clusters for the diagnostic profile: self-limiting features, underdeveloped behaviour and unsupported development. These have two, three and five sub-clusters, respectively. The latter two clusters have sub-clusters that relate to 'Attachment'.

The factors likely to affect the scores obtained include matters such as visual impairment, limited understanding of language, medical conditions or others which may affect the scores obtained from the first two parts of the profile.

Easterbrook (2006) finds the descriptions:

> very straightforward and specific making them easy to score. Grouping the answers into sub-clusters and clusters that are then interpreted appears to take care of the 'thinking', but planning an intervention consists only of samples. The visual representation in the histograms of the progress made by the case studies was impressive and the comparison to 'normal functioning' allows perspective. (p.15)

However, Easterbrook (2006) believes that the likelihood of the profile being completed only by a teacher makes it too subjective, although she does not doubt its usefulness in the classroom. Easterbrook adds that her understanding is that at the Mulberry Bush School the profile is completed, like the needs assessment, collectively, which would give it its strength in such a setting.

National Children's Bureau assessment model

The National Children's Bureau (NCB) created, through its care planning for looked-after children project, what has been called the needs-outcome-service model.[2] The model moves from identifying need to deciding what would occur if the need were met (outcome) to meeting the need (service) to reviewing what was done and what happened.

Kane (2007) describes the elements of each step. Need, she says, consists of what children require to thrive in terms of health and development and to meet their potential as they move towards adulthood and beyond. To establish whether need is met the practitioner has to decide what outcome is desired. A concept like the child being happy is too vague and is unrealistic because no human being can be happy all the time. Thus, outcomes need to be what Kane calls 'SMART': Specific, Measurable, Achievable, Realistic and Time-limited. Evidence must also be provided that the outcome has been achieved. A useful starting point is to define what the outcome will look like when it has been achieved, or how we will know when it has been achieved.

A service is whatever is needed – therapy, foster care, a residential placement, reunion with the family – to meet the need by performing specific tasks. So, for example, a foster carer listens to the child or a counselling service offers trauma counselling.

When the service or the task is evaluated to see if it met the need this is the review stage. If the need has not been met, a different service or task may be required. Kane (2007) also stresses that 'it is extremely important to record needs that have been identified and not been met or cannot be met and the reasons for this' (p.21).

Common Assessment Framework

The Common Assessment Framework was introduced in 2006. It was proposed in *Every Child Matters* (HM Treasury 2003) as another means of drawing professionals together and ensuring that information is shared, consistent and not lost, while reducing unnecessary duplication in assessment. The Green Paper (HM Treasury 2003) had pointed out that children may receive many assessments during their childhood: by health visitors; the baseline assessment in the first year of primary school; secondary schools, which are increasingly introducing individual learning plans; social services; Connexions; youth offending teams; education psychologists; and others.

The problems arising from several agencies and professionals recording information were exacerbated because, although the information may be similar (but not always, depending on the defined need at the time of a particular assessment), different professional terms and categories were employed. Added to this, the core information does not follow the child, so children and families are then asked to provide the same information several times to different people – and often still without a practical result.

The Department of Health and the Department for Education and Employment (2000) devised the 'assessment framework triangle' (Figure 1.1). This explains the areas which an assessment for a child in need should cover to create a holistic assessment.

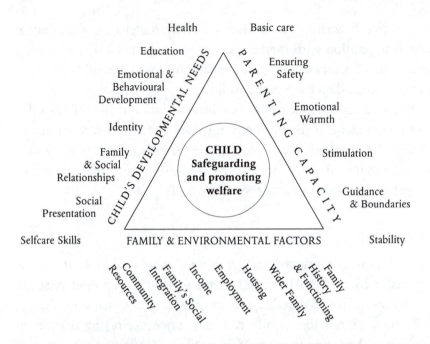

Figure 1.1 *Assessment framework triangle (from Department of Health and Department for Education and Employment 2000). © Crown copyright 2000. Reproduced under the terms of the Click-Use Licence.*

However, as Raynes (2006) points out, there is no common assessment framework for children 'in need' and 'at risk of significant harm' (in the terms of the Children Act 1989). Despite the recommendation of Lord Laming's inquiry into the death of Victoria Climbié (Laming 2003) that the guidance on the assessment framework and *Working Together to Safeguard Children* (DoH, Home Office and DfEE 1999) be combined, this has not been done. This means, for example, that the 15 days that child protection workers have to go to a case conference tallies ill with the 35 days they have to complete the core assessment for a child in need. This seems to militate against the contention of *Every Child Matters* (HM Treasury 2003) that 'child protection cannot be separated from policies to improve children's lives as a whole'. There are also children and young people's strategic partnerships now vying with local safeguarding boards with no indication of how they should work together, showing both symbolically and practically, the bifurcation between assessments for children in need and those at risk of significant harm.

This shows again how bureaucratic remedies do not fit the realities of the lives of children and their families.

Assessment, race and culture

An assessment must be made in light of an understanding of the child's race and culture by doing what Dalzell and Sawyer (2007) call 'a cultural review'. The purpose of this, they say:

> is for the practitioner to alert themselves [*sic*] to areas where their own assumptions, prejudices or simply lack of knowledge might have a bearing on their response to a family and, ultimately, on the approach taken to working with them. Similarly, issues that a worker may be carrying in their head, such as agency norms and awareness, will also have an impact. (p.18)

The need is for practitioners to be familiar with and understand the culture of those with whom they work and this knowledge cannot be overemphasized. All children have needs, some children have special needs and children from black and ethnic minorities have a set of needs arising from their origins. However, while it is important to recognize and act upon them so that the child is not doubly or even triply disadvantaged, this should not be done to the exclusion of all else. Just as no child should be seen as the sum total of her problems, so also no child should be seen as defined wholly from her racial or cultural background. If this happens, there is a real danger that other important factors, which are a part of the child's situation and her family's life and background, may be overlooked. Who she is will be partial and her needs distorted (Banks 2001). Part of this consideration is also a tendency to view culture in a way that is unhelpful, which Banks (2001) warns against. 'Culture is not static; it is an evolving dynamic within and between groups,' he says.

Race and culture are important. They do not dominate the life of a child, but ignoring them or misunderstanding them can be disastrous. Kane (2007) asks a number of questions that the practitioner should ask himself. For example, what he knows of children and families from a particular background or life experience, what is the source of his knowledge, what prejudices – negative or positive – does he harbour, how might the child and family see him, how might the agency and assessment be perceived, and what effect on the child and family could the assessment have? (p.18). Kane goes on to explain:

> As well as looking at the internal world of the child, considerations have to be given to the environment in which the child lives, past, present and future. There may be needs that have to be addressed as a result. There also has to be an awareness that looked-after children may face discrimination on many levels because of their ethnicity, culture, religion or beliefs, their gender, sexuality, age or because they are in the care system. (p.20)

The human factor

Lest it be thought that even with our emphasis on including the whole team, and not regarding assessment as a mechanistic, objective, scientific activity which we are placing our faith in, it must be said that assessment is carried out by people, by individuals. Not only should they not tick boxes and not only should they be properly trained, qualified and supervised, but they must bring essential human qualities to the task. Saying they will do what they say they will do, and being reliable, honest, non-judgemental, respectful, courteous, trustworthy, empathetic and open underwrites all else. Even the most perfectly devised assessment process will, at best, falter and, at worst, fail, if these qualities are not part and parcel of everything that the practitioner offers the child.

CHAPTER 2

Plans and Outcomes

The Green Paper, *Every Child Matters* (HM Treasury 2003) was specifically concerned with all children in all aspects of their lives. It said:

> Our aim is to ensure that every child has the chance to fulfil their potential by reducing levels of educational failure, ill health, substance misuse, teenage pregnancy, abuse and neglect, crime and anti-social behaviour among children and young people. (p.6)

The government consulted with children, young people and families 'to set out a positive vision of the outcomes' that it wanted to achieve. From this emerged five outcomes which mattered most to the children and young people themselves. These have now become the underpinning principles of children's services – health, education and social care – and apply to all children. But they are also helpful to bear in mind, especially when thinking about the needs of vulnerable, neglected and abused children, because they form a useful summary under which more detailed and specific outcomes may be placed or which can help lead us to them. The Green Paper (HM Treasury 2003) outcomes were:

- **being healthy**: enjoying good physical and mental health and living a healthy lifestyle

- **staying safe**: being protected from harm and neglect

- **enjoying and achieving**: getting the most out of life and developing the skills for adulthood

- **making a positive contribution**: being involved with the community and society, and not engaging in anti-social or offending behaviour

- **economic well-being**: not being prevented by economic disadvantage from achieving their full potential in life.

(pp.6–7)

Strengths and weaknesses of an outcomes-based approach

We began this book by saying that in the past decade or so there has been a shift in favour of *outcomes*. However, this has not avoided a damaging confusion between outcomes and inputs, almost as if they were interchangeable or that inputs themselves inevitably lead to better outcomes. Willis (2001) said, 'the major focus of quality initiatives over the past decade has not been on defining how these outcomes might be evaluated in practice, but on standards and measures of inputs, processes and outputs' (p.140). This may be because inputs, processes and *outputs* are easier to measure than outcomes, but concentration on inputs is unhelpful. For example, we can measure the number of visits which children make to the dentist, but that says nothing about the standard of the dental care or the health of the children's teeth. The number of children in care who attend school regularly speaks nothing of the quality of the education which they receive, nor does the number of children and young people with mental health problems having access to child and adolescent mental health services indicate what kind of service they get and, more important, what it achieves.

An output, then, is a measurement of process that can tell us only so much, and little, if anything at all, about what the service is like. In our own lives, none of us would be satisfied with an output because what we want for ourselves and our children are *outcomes*.

Writing in the last century, Rilke (1903) was not offering advice to the Department for Schools, Children and Families or the Department of Health when he wrote:

Don't search for the answers which cannot be given because you would not be able to live them. And life is about living every-thing. Live the questions now. Perhaps, then, gradually, without noticing it you'll live yourself into the answer.

However, this may be construed not as a counsel against setting targets, but more that we should not become dependent on them. Targets can, in fact, miss the point of what they are supposed to measure: is the final product of education to be only the acquisition of examination results and is a 'good' school to be judged only on how many of its pupils acquire so many results at this or that level? Education seen in the round is not inimical to academic success but it is also about how children adjust to one another, to a system of authority, to the acquisition of social skills and values and how they view the world.

As Harvey (2006) argues, education is not just about examination results and getting qualifications. It is part of a bigger, fluid and indi-vidual process, which ignites something within children and equips them with values and aspirations on which they build for the rest of their lives. The French, having grasped that education can go on throughout a person's life, coined the phrase 'education permanente': continuous and unending education.

In social care the tendency to 'tick the box' is now recognized as, equally, missing what is important about a service. For example, the Commission for Social Care Inspection has loosened its inspection regimen to make ticking boxes less important than finding out how those who use services experience them. The outcome here, as elsewhere, remains critical for, as Mabey (2005) rightly points out, 'in the nature of things life will always keep one step ahead of the measurers and managers' (p.126). And so to stay with the measurers will be to be one step behind life.

Outcomes have come comparatively late to social care as a way of determining the most appropriate ways of helping people. Willis (2001) talks about initiatives from the Department of Health in the 1990s founded on a statement by the Social Services Inspectorate in 1993:

> social care services are likely to be the most effective when they
> are orientated toward outcomes: concerned with, designed,
> provided and evaluated in terms of the results experienced by the
> people for whom they are intended. (p.193)

One of the most recent emphases on outcomes for children's services
came with the Children Act 2004, which requires children's agencies
not only to work toward the goals of the Green Paper (HM Treasury
2003) but to provide evidence about their achievement.

To define an outcome as a product, result or consequence, though,
is too broad for our purposes. Tomlinson (in press) suggests that it is
necessary, first, to narrow our focus to achieving positive outcomes,
and, second, that the outcome needs to be defined as positive by the
user of the service.

Outcomes have come to replace the more qualitative judgements
that have held sway in the past. In the field of therapy this has tended
to be about what kind of therapy was most appropriate, as if deciding
on appropriateness said anything about the end product – did the
therapy have any effect?

As Ball and colleagues (2004) write:

> There is a real danger that a focus on outcomes may be over-
> looked or simply paid lip service, while managers concentrate on
> more explicit and pressing requirements such as implementing
> the single assessment process, or bringing services in line with
> performance indicators. (p.13)

The irony of this is, of course, that the only way of knowing what
works effectively is by observing the outcome of the intervention.
And, as Ball and colleagues (2004) go on to say – perhaps somewhat
ironically given their reservations about the way managers work –
'people get excited about better outcomes; they don't get excited about
performance indicators'. They say that the evidence is that when the
concern for outcomes is what shapes services, performance indicators
look after themselves. Indicators can never tell the whole story and can
only be useful when used with other information, such as what users of
services say, other kinds of survey and looking at what complaints can

tell us. As Ball and colleagues (2004) baldly but correctly put it, 'performance indicators should do just what their name suggests – indicate'.

But outcomes themselves are not value free: they have to be analysed. Tomlinson (in press) advises that we measure 'equality outcomes', that is, to check that outcomes are achieved equally by all different groups – those of different race or gender for example – receiving the same service.

Ball and colleagues (2004) carried out research into the possible benefits of assessing outcomes as a part of practice. They reported several: the assessment process was more focused; attention was given to aspirations and not just problems; users' and carers' priorities were highlighted; there was greater recognition of carers; care plans were more creative and aimed specifically at the needs of individuals; there was clearer guidance about the purpose of help and what individuals needed from services providers; differences of outlook were clarified, which helped in negotiations; and how people felt about services helped to adjust care packages (p.15). This shows how it is possible to develop and improve services through a willingness to learn from the service user.

The idea of the learning organization has become, for at least one local authority, a wish to become an 'outcome-orientated organization'. North Lincolnshire has impressed Ball and colleagues (2004), who think that 'this idea has a life beyond the corporate froth of mission statements and glossy plans'. What this means, they say, is:

- how performance review systems have been designed

- the investment that has been made in information systems which help staff manage and judge critical processes that contribute to better outcomes

- how processes of assessment, planning and review are designed

- the expectation of user involvement in decision-making

- the emphasis given to outcomes in the staff training programme

- willingness to engage in action research on outcomes with academic institutions and others.

(p.16)

Sense and assessment

Children who have been abused and neglected suffer from deficiencies in their experience of parenting or the lack of it. The task of assessment is to identify what these deficiencies are, and so this will take place early in the placement.

We have quoted Ward (2004) earlier, but it is worth here reiterating that he refers to assessment as a:

> process of making sense of current available experience, to help you have some idea of what is going on in your interactions with the child, in order that you may modify, interrupt, emphasize or even ignore certain aspects of the dynamic. (p.9)

Assessment gathers essential information about the child and understands her current experience, and this must be informed by a thorough and detailed knowledge of a child's history and previous experience.

By looking into the child's past the source of her trauma can be identified. We can also discover which basic needs were met and which were not, and what may have affected her development. Stages of the child's development can be outlined, and we can also know what developmental milestones have been achieved and which ones missed. We can also identify what abuse and neglect may have occurred. Her history may tell us how she is likely to respond to new carers, as well as providing clues about how she perceives what is happening to her now. Knowing her past may also allow us to know what events may trigger strong feelings and responses, as well as identifying how she has coped with stress in the past (Pughe and Philpot 2007).

It is critical when making an assessment to know how a child's mind works. Fahlberg (1994) sums this up succinctly:

Children, particularly young children, believe that their lives are 'normal'. They are incapable of comparing their own situation with that of others. They incorporate their own experiences into their overall view of what family life is like and take these perceptions and their own reactions to them into any new settings. (p.232)

Patterns, too, will appear as a result of investigation: behaviour patterns and those which have precipitated placement; the significance of anniversaries and incidents, and recreations of a situation or relationship from the child's past. We will come to know about her education, as well as how she has coped socially, for example when she has lived in groups. The family history may identify family patterns, scripts and the history of relationships with others (Rose and Philpot 2005).

SACCS has developed an assessment process that draws together these essential elements of past and present and gives priority to the sharing of information and insights that each element may provide. Current information and experience is taken from all three areas of the recovery team, thus integrating therapeutic parenting, life story and therapy (*see* Chapter 4).

Assessment may be seen as a chart of how far a child has journeyed on the road to recovery. But such a map requires us to define what destination we hope she will reach and how to know when she has reached it.

The desired outcomes

Twenty-four outcomes have been set which recognize that recovery has been achieved. If a child is able to demonstrate she is reaching these outcomes it is felt she would most likely have reached the point of recovery as described.

The outcomes comprise a child who:

- **has a sense of self of whom she is and where she has been.** This means that the child has a sense of her own identity and culture, regardless of creed, race, nationality, or religion, especially if there are also issues of disability and/or gender. She understands about her family of origin, has worked through what she loves, hates, is angry about, is frightened of, and is not in denial. She knows who she is in relationship to important people in her past and significant people in her present. She has integrated her past experiences into her present reality. Her personality is clear and intact. The child is living mostly in the present. Her past is no longer controlling her life.

- **has an understanding of her past history and experiences.** That is she has thoroughly worked through the issues and trauma in her past and has understood what has happened to her, when and in what order with her current cognitive ability. The child has some insights how her past experiences impact on her present behaviour. Her internal working model of the world has expanded to incorporate new models of how to be.

- **is able to show appropriate reactions.** She can recognize her feelings accurately and her behaviour is able to convey that feeling to others, so that she feels sad and doesn't laugh, or feels frightened and doesn't put herself into more dangerous situations, or feels angry and wants to be loving. She is able to feel love and be loving, feel the pain and be sad, feel rage and be angry, and feel frightened and be scared.

- **has developed internal controls** and thus is able to recognize what is right and what is wrong and wants to regulate her behaviour herself within what is considered acceptable. External controls, boundaries and supervision no longer have to be so intense, and the child has built up a level of trust with her carers, and is confident that she will be able to contain her feelings and behaviour.

- **is able to make use of opportunities** so that she is no longer a victim of the world, but is now a survivor, recognizing possibilities and opportunities when they arise and is able to put herself forward to take advantage of those possibilities. It also means being able to ask for what she wants. It does not mean using opportunities to overwhelm and victimize other children, or to break the law in any other way.

- **is able to make appropriate choices** so that she is no longer a victim and able to recognize that she has choices available to her and that she is actually already exercising those choices. She is able to see that she has a future and can have an active role in shaping it, which can take a number of different forms. It also means that the choices that the child is able to make promote physical and emotional health.

- **is able to make appropriate adult and peer relationships.** She is able to recognize that she is a child of appropriate chronological age and is able to function at that age. The relationships and attachments that the child is able to make are appropriate to the situation. She is able to recognize that past relationships have been distorted through abusive or neglectful experiences.

- **is making academic progress** so that she is able to achieve her potential within her intellectual ability. It may mean that as the child becomes clearer, she is, therefore, better able to concentrate and to perform more productively within the range of ability. She is more able to get totally involved in tasks in the present, for example reading a story, and less involved with ruminating about negative things in the past.

- **is able to take responsibility** and is no longer in denial about her past. She apportioned blame appropriately and if it is part of her story is able to see her part in what happened. Taking responsibility implies being able to make choices, and being aware of them and any consequences that may occur as a result of that particular choice being made. Therefore the child is able to make a decision about what is to happen, knowing and accepting the result whatever it might be.

- **has developed conscience** and, thus, a sense of right and wrong, and is able to feel remorse if she has hurt someone or something. This can only be done in the context of a significant and safe relationship or attachment.

- **is no longer hurting herself or others.** This means that she is not physically, sexually, verbally, emotionally or intellectually victimizing other children or adults. Nor is she harming herself, physically, sexually, verbally, emotionally or intellectually. She recognizes that she is a valuable human being worthy of respect, and prepared to be respectful. She also understands that animals are not objects of physical or sexual torture or harm.

- **is developing insights.** Through an understanding of her past experiences, when it no longer has any power over her behaviour, thoughts and feelings; only then is the child able to see objectively who she is, and who significant others are, in relationship to her. Importantly, she is able to see her victimization not as something which she made happen, but rather the person who victimized her actively planned; she just happened to be there. She is then able to see the role of whatever adults were involved either in harming her or not protecting her or both.

- **has completed important developmental tasks.** When a child has been traumatized through abuse, she is sometimes 'pseudo-mature', or a preoccupation with the abusive relationship means that important developmental tasks have not been completed. The child will need to revisit these stages and ages in order to complete these tasks successfully so that she is able emotionally to grow up and achieve self-mastery. It also means that the adults around her are prepared to allow her to be the age she is now, to regress if needed to an earlier developmental stage, to acknowledge that and support it, and to help the child feel safe enough to do this work, and respect and affirm its importance.

- **has developed cause and effect thinking** so that she understands that when she does something there is a consequence, good, bad or indifferent. This implies that the child is able to make choices and to see that other people and other people's feelings and possessions matter. It also implies that she is able to think logically, and linearly, and is not egocentric.

- **understands sequences.** The child understands not only about cause and effect, and her part in it, but also about how one thing follows on from another, or leads to it and why. She is able to see links in a set of circumstances and a logical understanding of why this happens.

- **has developed motor skills** whereby she has met all her developmental milestones. She is less self-absorbed and much more aware of the space she has taken up in the world and her relationship to it. She is also much more able to concentrate on tasks, and be less lost in the past.

- **has developed abstract thinking** so that she is able to conceptualize without the object being in front of her. This is also an ability to represent symbolically her experience and distress and to get resolution through these symbolic representations.

- **has improved physical health** because she is receiving sufficient care and nurture, and safety. Her body and her spirit are able to recover their full potential.

- **has normal sleeping habits.** She will understand that going to sleep is a healthy, safe, necessary and lovely thing to do and doing this at the proper time is a prerequisite to normal functioning. The child does not have to be responsible for ensuring she has a safe night's sleep. She understands, too, that the rest of the world also sleeps at that time, which creates an understanding that there is time for everything: there will be a time for all her needs to be met. Structure and routine, being imposed by adults who care about them, is the beginning of relationship and/or attachment.

- **has normal personal hygiene.** She will have sufficient respect for herself that she wants to look after her body and bodily functions in the best way that she can. We need to understand that when traumatized children do not care for themselves, soil, smear or wet themselves, they are actually showing their pain, and not being disgusting, but rather showing us how disgusting they think they are. Traumatized children learn that their bodies are not worthy of respect or care and that means that they themselves are not worthy of respect or care. Adults who keep them safe, care and nurture them are able to teach them how to love and respect themselves within a trusting relationship.

- **has normal eating behaviours,** which means that she no longer has to overeat or refuse food for reasons linked to her past abuse, or either to comfort herself or harm herself. She may lack the skills to feed appropriately, and will learn these through a safe and loving relationship.

- **has normal body language,** which means that she develops awareness of how she is using her body to communicate to adults and those of her own age. This implies that she is aware of her own feelings and knows how to show them appropriately. It also means that she understands about acceptable touching, and her personal space and that of others. It is an awareness of what kind of touch is acceptable and loving, and what is not. It is an ability to use the language of their bodies, and to know what she is communicating to others.

- **has normal self-image.** She is able to acknowledge that she is as she is. She sees herself as others see her. She can acknowledge her strengths as well as being realistically aware of her weaknesses. The abused child carries a mental picture which is an image in her mind of her body which may be distorted as a result of past trauma. She is aware of the space she takes up in the world and her relatedness to everything around her. It is only when she can see herself through the eyes of significant people who love her that she can start to love herself.

- **is able to make positive contributions:** to respect herself and her opinions as a creative force. She is able to ask for what she wants, and intervenes appropriately in a positive way in other interactions. She is able to view the world as a healthy, safe and exciting place that she has a part in creating and influencing.

(Walsh 2002)

These outcomes are grouped together under six developmental areas:

- learning
- physical development
- emotional development
- attachment
- identity
- social and communicative development.

All of the outcomes are closely connected to fundamental human needs for safety, happiness and development. To assist practitioners in their aim to help children achieve the outcomes, the SACCS' recovery programme shows that each outcome is accompanied by series of tasks to achieve it, and each task has guidance on how it can be done. For example, for improved physical health, there are eight tasks. One of these is to ensure that personal hygiene needs are met in a caring and loving way, so that the child learns that caring for her body is part of loving herself. Another task is that the house will be run on healthy routines so that children are able to relax into boundaries and predictable timetables. This is especially important for chaotic children as it gives them a sense of security and of being anchored. Building in anchor points, routines and limits is necessary to enable each house to hold children emotionally, contain their anxiety and give appropriate opportunity for individual choice and autonomy.

For the first of these tasks the guidance is to:

- understand the child's history and, in particular, her formative experience in relation to hygiene

- use the recovery assessment to understand the child's stage of development, and what has been the impact of trauma on this and her physical well-being

- formulate a plan, as part of the therapeutic parenting team, to meet the child's personal hygiene needs in a caring and loving way, while taking account of the difficulties that might be involved (for example, being sensitive to the child's feelings of shame about intimate care)

- ensure that all daily routines about the child's personal care – washing, bathing, cleaning her teeth, combing her hair, nail cutting – are done reliably and consistently

- reflect the importance of personal care in the home by making sure that there is an emphasis on enjoyment in a child-centred way (for example, by providing bath toys and bubble baths)

- work closely with the recovery team so that everyone is aware of what is happening for the child.

It is important that such guidance is treated with concern for the individual child and her needs. These will differ from child to child, and each child is a complex person with a complicated history and set of experiences. Even where experiences are similar, reactions and needs will differ from child to child.

Pughe and Philpot (2007) summarize the SACCS' outcomes by saying that they are about:

> the child having internalized her attachments and consolidated her emotional development to the point where these can be successfully transferred to other environment and relationships. The child is then deemed to have the potential to achieve full ability in all aspects of her life. (p.112)

As well as gathering as much as possible of the child's current and previous details for an informed assessment, it is perhaps just as important how this information is brought together, shared and then used. As we have said, an assessment which is not only shared but created by all those with some responsibility for the child presents a holistic picture of her (*see* Chapter 4).

'A hierarchy of outcomes'

All of the outcomes just mentioned are broad and, ultimately, achievable, but they are maximum outcomes. To achieve them we need to adopt what Sawyer (2005) calls 'a hierarchy of outcomes', distinguishing between maximum and minimum outcomes. The maximum outcome is what Sawyer (2005) calls the over-arching outcome, and progress towards that may best be managed in a series of 'bite-sized outcomes' or minimum outcomes. A minimum outcome is not a second-best, it is a step or a series of steps towards the maximum. Perhaps this is what Dockar-Drysdale (1993) means when she talks about ditching the concept of 'cure' in favour of 'evolvement'.

Let us take some examples. If a child shows aggressive, even violent behaviour, the maximum outcome is that her relationship with others means that she does not act in that way. A step in that direction might be to seek a minimum outcome whereby, for example, she manages to get through a day without hurting anyone or swearing at them or otherwise acting aggressively.

Another example is that a child should ultimately be able to take responsibility. This may be so big a step that the child cannot even conceive of it. However, what may be understandable and achievable and a taking of responsibility is that she is able to help set the table for tea.

Independence for a child is another over-arching outcome, and this could be realized (to take the example given by Sawyer (2005)) by her making a simple meal, dressing and undressing without help, washing and showering on her own and organizing her own needs when shopping. Sawyer (2005) points out:

> Not only is this more likely to give the individual a more rapid sense of achievement, but also it will enable staff to focus on specific areas. (p.22)

There are other small but important steps. For example, a child might be able to be helped to go to bed without becoming unsettled, or she might communicate with a parent, or when a parent visits she can boast that she has learnt to ride a bike or tie her shoelaces. These are incremental achievements, small things which are tangible and so important to a child. A child's long-term prospects may be daunting and it may take hundreds of small steps to achieve them; children may also be encouraged to make their own goals and take their own steps.

In working with children in this way we are also helping them to make choices. But, again, choices can seem overwhelming, especially to a very traumatized child. To ask a child to choose what she wants to wear may be beyond her, but to offer her the choice of, say, one or two dresses is a choice she can make.

Helping children to achieve minimum outcomes on the way to achieving maximum ones is also about working at the pace that a child is able to cope with.

As Harvey (2006) says:

> We can let people develop at their own speed without hurrying them on simply because they have reached a particular age or stage. Hurry is not nourishing. It will not lead to true learning. Our hurrying a person on without taking into account his or her emotional and other sorts of readiness could be harmful, could delay his or her emotional growth. (p.148)

What makes a good plan?

It could be argued that the concentration on indicators rather than outcomes is related to some people saying that they have no time to plan. This makes no sense. If we do not think, we cannot plan, and if we do not plan we cannot act effectively. But the statement seems also to indicate that too often action is taken on the hoof, or instinctively. If the response to saying that that isn't the way to do things is, 'It's OK for you, you have the time' that leads only to poor services. To do something badly or ineffectively is worse, in many ways, than doing nothing at all. In services where costs are frequently cited, it is also a waste of money; in a service that works with people, at best, it delays finding the right course of action to help them; at worst, it damages them or makes their situation worse. In the long run, correctly organized assessment can be a way to create proper planning, aided by reflection, and it militates against seeking short-term measures or applying sticking plaster and will give better value for money. It also allows anticipation and *forward* planning. So, for someone to say that they do not have time to plan can never be valid and is more likely to be an excuse suggesting the practitioner has no idea what should be done.

Kane (2007) says that a good plan must be:

- explicit (all steps completely spelled out)

- intelligible (capable of being understood by all those who will carry it out)

- flexible (capable of accepting change)

- written (committed to writing in a clear, concise manner).

(p.16)

A good and a bad plan may be seen in terms of opposites. For example, a good plan is based on the needs of the service user; a bad plan is service-led. A child participates fully in a good plan which she understands. She is not only excluded in a bad plan but she does not understand it. Similarly, parents, those with parental responsibility and carers participate in a good plan; in bad planning they are given no part. A good plan, as we have said, is SMART (Specific, Measurable, Achievable, Realistic and Time-limited). The bad plan is unspecific about who does what; it has outcomes which cannot be evaluated; it is not achievable or realistic; and it has no timescale. Good plans have focus and are proactive; bad ones lack direction and are reactive. A good plan brings other plans together and also allows for contingencies but a bad one is separate from other plans and makes no allowance for contingencies (Kane 2007, p.17).

Another aspect of the good plan is that it draws in other plans, including the care plan, the personal education plan, the health plan and the placement plan. Older children will also have transition plans (where the child has a disability) and pathway plans. For those children with communication problems there will also be a communications plan.

It is worth pointing out that while the 'care plan' may be an all-purpose plan for all manner of plans drawn up by homes, schools and other agencies, there can only be one real care plan: the looked-after children (LAC) plan. Kane (2007) offers the definition by Williams and McCann (2006) of a LAC plan, which:

> determines why it is in the child's best interest to become looked after or whether support services would be able to meet their needs; it identifies their assessed needs and the services to meet

those needs; and sets out the framework for the services provided to the child and family to enable the desired goals and outcomes to be achieved. (p.8)

The care plan, which all looked-after children must have, together with health and personal education plans, must include the child's needs and how they will be met, the services to be provided, the type and detail of the proposed placement and the support in that placement, arrangements for contact and/or reunification with the child's family, arrangements for education and healthcare, the aims, desired outcomes and timescales, what action is to be taken and by whom, and contingency plans (Kane 2007, p.9).

Health plans include arrangements for health assessments by a qualified medical practitioner (although this can be carried out by a designated nurse) to create the health plan.

The pathway plan is for children aged over 16 and builds on the care plan and other plans; it becomes the care plan for the young person when they reach the age to leave care.

Placement plans are written plans for the child's daily life in placement and detail how the child will be looked after and how her needs will be met by the carer or residential home.

CHAPTER 3

Understanding the Whole Child

When a child is being assessed, recognition has to be given to what developmental stage she has reached: What should she be expected to be able to do? What skills is she capable of? How should she be expected to act and react? What behaviour and language are appropriate to her age? Child development is a series of stages through which a child passes from dependent infancy and childhood through adolescence to autonomous, interdependent adulthood. This process involves a number of changes – physical, cognitive, emotional, behavioural, social and educational – during which the child is both learning from the world she inhabits and comes to be conscious of the fact that she inhabits it. It explains how children act at certain times and may be plotted by observing certain developmental milestones, a clear understanding of which are essential to assessment.

A child who is loved and safe and made to feel secure should develop healthily. However, things can occur in this developmental journey – for infant, small child and adolescent – which can impede and, in some cases, set back or arrest a healthy development. Such events in a child's life can range from the mother's experience when pregnant to serious accident, bereavement and physical, mental or sexual abuse.

Quoting the marital therapist and writer Jack Dominion, Harvey (2006) says that maturity is:

> The cohering of our intellectual, social, cultural, spiritual and
> emotional sides into one integrated 'system' which enables us to
> give love to others, to go out to them in trust and affection, and to
> accept them as they are. (p.22)

Ward (1996) refers to 'seven key developmental dimensions: health, education, identity, family and social relationships, social presentation, emotional and behavioural development, and self-care skills' (p.243). Thus, the child's development is shaped by a number of factors, including her relationship with her parents (in particular, her mother) or primary caregiver, and her relationship with others (initially her family and gradually those in the world outside of it, particularly, early on, with other children). Her genetic inheritance will also determine her development, as will nutrition and the quality of education (and early learning, pre-school and her interaction in the early years with her parents). Race, gender, religion, culture, age and disability will shape how she sees herself and conceives of her own identity and, importantly, the reaction of others to her.

That said, each child is different and assessments must recognize those nuances, differences and factors that intermingle with the commonalities which all children share, as the Department of Health and the Department for Education and Employment (2000) emphasize:

> Each child's development is significantly shaped by his or her
> particular experiences and the interaction between a series of
> factors. Some factors are intrinsic to individual children, such as
> characteristics of inheritance or temperament. Other factors may
> include particular health problems or an impairment. Others may
> relate to their culture and to the physical and emotional environ-
> ment in which a child is living. (p.11)

For children with disabilities, especially perhaps those with a learning disability, there may be different rates of progress during development. Some of these children may work at different paces; for example, a child with autism may have acquired some skills in advance of the milestones but other skills, such as communication, may be non-existent. At different ages, too, different emphases apply: for the young child it is about acquiring cognitive and language skills, whereas the teenager 'strives to reconcile the tensions between social and emotional dependence and independence' (DoH and DfEE 2000, p.36).

This statement goes on to emphasize that professionals should understand the various consequences for the particular ages of children. Plans and assessments should be based on the child's development progress at different stages or milestones and action taken, when necessary, that is 'timely and appropriate in terms of the child's developmental needs' (DoH and DfEE 2000, p.11).

Attachment

Attachment is a theory about behaviour, bonds, relationships and reactions to loss and fear. It is about our sense of self and our empathetic connection to others. It is also a theory of developmental psychopathology. It raises questions about how one manages oneself under stressful and threatening circumstances, whether they are physical or psychological. What are the strategies, conscious and unconscious, which one adopts in the face of a perceived threat and what are the consequences?

Attachment theory has become critical in the understanding and healing of severely traumatized children. Kennell, Voos and Klaus (1976) defines attachment as 'an affection bond between two individuals that endures through space and time and serves to join them emotionally'. Howe (2000) explains that 'attachment behaviour is an instinctive biological drive that propels infants into protective proximity with their main carers whenever they experience anxiety, fear or distress' (p.26). When attachment has never been formed or severed or fractured, the task of recovery is to create or restore it.

The theory is commonly associated with John Bowlby (1973–1980), although others have added to his work.[3] Bowlby (1953) came to the conclusion that 'when deprived of maternal care, a child's development is almost always retarded – physically, intellectually and socially – and that symptoms of physical and mental illness may appear' (p.21). However, all ideas are based on close observation and work has been carried out on the effects of loss and separation experienced by children evacuated during the Second World War.[4] This means that attachment disorder is not something which only affects children severely traumatized by abuse. It seeks to explain why patterns of behaviour either persist or change, over time and across relationships.

When first formulated attachment theory emphasized the parent–child relationship, and whilst that relationship remains formative, it is now also known that other relationships throughout our lives can have an impact on our attachment. Children who have suffered long periods of separation from their parents or who have lost their parents and suffered severe emotional difficulties can find it extremely difficult to make relationships with others and can become withdrawn. They can exhibit other various kinds of behaviour problems. Thus, a nurturing and loving relationship allows us to develop maturely and make healthy relationships with others. For the purposes of this book we are looking at the most extreme disruption of attachment, so that if the relationship is violent and involves rejection, pain, abuse, lack of bonding and disruption, then it is very likely that the child will be unable to relate healthily to others and form loving and trusting relationships. There is then the possibility that there may be problems, such as criminal, violent or abusive sexual behaviour. Of course, anxiety, loss and distress are integral to our lives but sufficient emotional resilience, which lack of attachment destroys or impairs, is crucial to facing and dealing with them.

Levy and Orlans (1998) note another characteristic of at least some abused children who have attachment disorders. They 'have an inordinate need for punitive and/or coercive control of others', which militates against a rapport with their carers. Levy and Orlans (1998) go on to call these children 'extremely emotionally defensive' who, while experiencing sadness, worthlessness, rejection and fear, 'generally only allow for the expression of anger. They feel empowered by demonstrations of anger and aggression'. They continue:

They learn at an early age that anger works: if others retreat in response to their anger, they believe they have won; if others escalate in response to their provocation, they also believe they have won, because they have engaged others 'on their terms'. Certain caregiver or therapist responses, such as anger, helplessness or emotional distance, serve to empower the child's negative patterns... (pp.116–117)

It should be emphasized, though, that while attachment is formed in the early days, weeks and months of a child's life, its lack can be witnessed in adults in their personal and sexual relationships and in their role as parents. The extreme behaviours we have just referred to – crime and violent and abusive sexual behaviour – may show in children but may also carry on into adult life.

Attachment theory propounds a blueprint called the 'internal working model', which is created for each of us in the early months of life. It is the mechanism through which the child attempts to connect herself, other people and the relationship between them. The quality of the child's caring experiences will determine whether the internal working model is positive or negative.

Levy and Orlans (1998) explain the internal working model as:

the cognitive representation of early attachment relationships. Based on attachment patterns with primary caregivers (e.g., secure, avoidant, ambivalent, disorganized), children develop beliefs and expectations about themselves, others and life in general: 'I am good/bad, lovable/unlovable, competent/helpless; caregivers are responsive/unresponsive, trustworthy/untrustworthy, caring/hurtful; the world is safe/unsafe; life is worth living/not worth living'. These early attachment experiences become internalized as core beliefs and anticipatory images that influence their later perceptions, emotions and reactions to others (e.g., foster and adoptive parents). (p.46)

The quality of the child's caring experiences will determine whether the internal working model is positive or negative. The attachment categories, to which Levy and Orlans (1998) have just referred, are widely recognized and have a major influence on the development of the child's internal working model:

- **secure attachment** (the carer is loving and the child is loved)

- **ambivalence** (the caregiver is inconsistent in how he responds and the child sees herself as dependant and poorly valued)

- **avoidant** (the caregiver is seen as consistently rejecting and the child is insecure but compulsively self-reliant)

- **disorganized** (caregivers are seen as frightening or frightened and the child is helpless, or angry and controlling).

(Howe 2000)

The last response is one often associated with children who have been maltreated. Levy and Orlans (1998) talk about the 'negative working model' to emphasize the disruption to the healthy internal working model, which they see as 'new belief system…the establishment of which is a primary goal of treatment' (p.117).

'Road maps' are what Archer (2003) calls internal working models. They provide, she says, children with another world, which Perry (1999) calls 'experience-dependent'. According to Burnell and Archer (2003) this framework:

maps out the most suitable response-routes to familiar, and unfamiliar challenges. IWMs [internal working models] reflect the child's view of, and confidence in, the attachment figures' capacity to provide a safe and caring environment. Moreover, these models, in turn, organize the child's thoughts, memories and feelings regarding attachment figures. Inevitably, they will also act as guides and predictors of future behaviour for the child and analogous attachment figures, such as adoptive parents. (p.65)

Schore (1994) describes these models as being burned into the unconscious at the neurobiological level, and Solomon and George (1999) say that, once established, they are highly resistant to change.

The implications and the consequences of a lack of attachment, loss, separation and abuse can be profound and far-reaching. They can affect how a child relates to her foster carer, social worker, teacher, friends and family, even strangers. She can fail to engage with school and the community. Children who experience a number of placements in care (a very common situation) can undergo a double loss – that of a sense of belonging in terms of relationships and also of place as they may be situated hundreds of miles from their home, community and family.

The psychological damage suffered by such children is immense, but inextricably interwoven with this can be the neurobiological damage that we now know can result from abuse and violence. At one time neurological and psychoanalytical explanations were regarded as inimical to one another. But it is no longer a matter of 'either/or' but rather of 'and/both' if we are to understand the many ways in which human beings react to trauma as well as recover from it. Thus, we now know that the forces of nurture and nature are much more intertwined than was previously imagined. This interferes with the growth of the brain and this damage manifests itself externally in various forms of disturbed behaviour (Perry 1999).

Levy and Orlans (1998) claim that:

> Modifying the negative working model is a major treatment goal with children with attachment disorder. This is extremely difficult, however, because these core beliefs become fixed, rigid, operate outside of conscious awareness, and do not often change as a result of modifying the child's environment... Placing such a child in a loving foster or adoptive home may only serve to exacerbate the problem. The child will push the love away due to lack of trust, expectation of maltreatment, and an unconscious attempt to recreate prior negative attachment patterns. (p.47)

When intervention with a child succeeds in creating a secure attachment and 'an autonomous internal working model', then, according to Prior and Glaser (2006) this:

> enables the child to move flexibly between seeking and receiving comfort and protection and free exploration, as circumstances require. There is now firm evidence indicating that a move toward security can be, and most effectively, achieved by enhancing the maternal/caregiver sensitivity expressed by the mother's behaviour with the child. (p.267)

Cairns (2002) explains that when parenting is negative (and this may affect children who are understimulated, let alone those whose parents abuse them) some brain connections are not produced and there is 'pruning' of connections already existing but unused. She asserts that there is a 'qualitative difference' between the brains of the securely attached child and the child who is unattached. Indeed, Cairns (2002) says, securely attached children develop bigger brains:

> Confronted with persistent unresolved stress, the infant brain forms characteristic user-dependent structures of either hyper-arousal or defensive association: hyper-aroused infants show perpetual signs of distress and irritability, while dissociated infants show none despite being in a physiological state of high arousal. (p.50)[5]

Perry and Szalavitz (2006) say that the brain changes in response to 'patterned repetitive experiences [such as basic primary care]: the more you repeat something, the more engrained it becomes'. They continue:

> This means that because it takes time to accumulate repetitions, recovery takes time and patience is called for as these repetitions continue. The longer the period of trauma, or the more extreme the trauma, the greater the number of repetitions required to regain balance. (p.245)

It is becoming more and more recognized that even babies may develop mental health problems as a result of early abuse. This is explained by YoungMinds (2004):

The vulnerability of babies and toddlers to mental health problems is increasingly acknowledged. The effect of these problems on subsequent functioning – physical, cognitive and emotional – is being investigated widely. Research strongly suggests that the way in which the brain develops is linked to early infant relationships, most often with the primary carer. Whilst other relationships in later life can be crucial, for example relationships with adoptive parents, these primary infant/carer relationships have a key impact on the mentally healthy development of the child...

Effects of trauma

Trauma is defined by Ziegler (2002) as 'anything that disrupts the optimal development of a child'. There are many things which can have this effect: a very difficult birth, a mother being physically abused when she is pregnant or a mother's smoking, drinking alcohol and taking drugs when pregnant. Poor care in pregnancy and the mother's emotional instability can also have negative effects on the foetus. A child may also be severely affected by separation from her mother, her mother's lack of interest in her or a father's absence or lack of support.

It is not difficult to see that severe physical, mental, emotional or sexual abuse (and, most commonly, a combination of two or more of these) will have devastating effects on a child. Neither does a child have to be beaten about the head for her brain to be affected. Neural pathways can also be affected by other forms of physical abuse, as well as by neglect and sexual abuse.

Ziegler (2002) says that 'the most serious finding' of the past decade is that neglect has the most long-lasting effect on development and is the 'most persistent and pervasive' form of trauma. According to him:

> The concern is not only how the brain reacts to neglect as a threat to survival, but also what the brain is *not* doing while preoccupied in survival mode. Neglect shifts the focus of the infant away from

the exploration and essential learning the brain is prepared to do
at the beginning of life. (p.37)

But children, no less than the rest of us, are individuals and respond
differently to different events. It is, therefore, wise to bear in mind that
while *all* trauma has a negative effect, *some* kinds of trauma affect *some*
children in *different* ways and that this will depend on the type of
trauma, the age of the child and the circumstances in which she was in
at the time it happened, and the resilience of the child. As James (1994)
explains:

> Psychological trauma occurs when an actual or perceived threat
> of a danger overwhelms a person's usual coping ability. Many sit-
> uations that are generally highly stressful to children might not
> be traumatizing to a particular child; some are able to cope and,
> even if the situation is repeated or chronic, are not developmen-
> tally challenged. The diagnosis of traumatization should be based
> on the context and meaning of the child's experience, not just on
> the event alone. What may appear to be a relatively benign expe-
> rience from an adult perspective – such as a child getting 'lost' for
> several hours during a family outing – can be traumatizing to a
> youngster. Conversely, a child held hostage with her family at
> gunpoint might not comprehend the danger and feel relatively
> safe. (pp.10–11)

James' use of the word 'overwhelming' is literally true. Trauma, in the
clinical sense, is far more devastating and means more than its popular
meaning of a bad shock. Its effects may be, at times, uncontrollable.
They may, literally, include helplessness, vulnerability to the point of a
fear for one's life, experiencing a loss of safety so that one feels wary of
others and a loss of control so that one's actions become unpredictable.

Trauma can affect a child's sense of identity, development, trust in
others, their ability to manage their behaviour and so on. Some adults
may feel this, too: from the man who is tortured in war to the woman
who is brutally raped. Because of her vulnerability a child, however,
may be affected by trauma in a much more far-reaching way and her

general social and individual functioning may well be seriously impaired.

Children who have suffered deeply as a result of trauma may experience a problem with memory: it may be suppressed or distorted or, on the other hand, crystal clear and intrusive so that the traumatic incident is continually remembered in all its detail.

One way that children try to cope with this is through 'magical thinking', of which Fahlberg (1994) says:

> For the preschool child it is their magical and egocentric thinking that most affects the reaction to parent loss. These children think they caused the loss, and that it came about because of their wishes, thoughts or behaviours. Their propensity for magical thinking is usually reinforced by a loss and is, therefore, likely to persist long beyond the age at which it commonly subsides.
>
> Adults hold responsibility for trying to identify the specific magical thinking of the child they are working with or parenting. What does the child think he/she did that caused the move? Or what could the child have done to prevent it? What does he/she think could be done to have the desired outcome? These are questions the adult, not the child, must answer. (p.138)

Fahlberg (1994) continues that magical thinking sometimes:

> takes place on an unconscious basis, particularly when it reflects the 'good vs bad' or the 'big vs little' struggles so commonly associated with this developmental stage [preschool years]. Behaviours may provide clues to the child's misperceptions. Carers, both before and after the move, should listen for comments that seem to make no sense, noting any odd or peculiar statements or behaviours. If carefully examined, these frequently give clues as to this child's perceptions and magical thinking. (p.138)

Fahlberg (1994) is talking about those children making the 'journey through placement' but they are equally applicable to other severe and far-reaching disruptions suffered by children.

Magical thinking is a way children fill in the gaps in their knowledge. When they don't know, they make it up. For example, a foster placement breaks down and the child is moved to a new home but why did the breakdown happen? If the child blames herself for the breakdown (as she may well do), then she will conclude the same again when the next breakdown occurs (as well it might). It is safer for the child to believe this but it only adds to her confusion about why she is where she is. The effect of this is carried through life – children who have filled the gaps in their own lives with their own fantasies, theories and stories do not become adults who are suddenly apprised of the truth. Life-story work helps to give meaning to magical thinking, of why children have believed what they have believed to be the truth about their lives, and to understand distortion, and allows them to confront their demons (Rose and Philpot 2005) (*see* Chapter 4).

Children who have been abused are also very likely to have a confused view of family relationships (Rose and Philpot 2005), as well as an ever-changing group of people in their lives, which, ironically, is not diminished when they go into care given the strong possibility of them being placed with a variety of foster carers, residential placements and a changing round of social workers.

Fahlberg (1994) says that one of the functions of family:

> is to provide continuous contact with a small number of people over a lifetime. The long-term relationships between family members allow each person an opportunity to clarify past events and reinterpret past events in terms of the present. Children in care are frequently denied these opportunities. They change families; they change workers; they may lose contact with birth family members.

Such events lead to children feeling that they lack control over their lives. The child's attempted solution to this problem can have disastrous consequences, for example by becoming suicidal or, at very least, self-harming and self-abusing by taking drugs or engaging in promiscuous and potentially harmful sexual relationships. The child may develop serious antisocial behaviour to defend her against vulnerability, but which actually exacerbates her difficulties.

Children will often revert to a state of helplessness. They can (like adults) adapt so that, for example, they avoid intimacy, feel that they need to be in control and act in ways that deter relationships and closeness with others. They can experience flashbacks, hyperactivity and dissociation. These, in turn, can affect their education and lead them to be diagnosed with various behavioural disorders.

James (1994) lists the four major effects of trauma on children as: a persistent state of fear, disordered memory, avoiding intimacy and 'dysregulation of affect'.[6] Dissociation – when painful and traumatic events are presented with an absence of emotion or appropriate emotion – is another consequence of trauma. It is what Hunter (2001) calls 'an internal psychological state which we assume is present when a usual or expected involvement of emotion is absent' (p.98).

Trauma can also have a very serious effect on attachment (*see below*). Ziegler (2002) refers to one reaction to trauma when he says:

> For traumatized individuals, emotions have lost their usefulness in providing important information to the reasoning centers of the neocortex, and emotions become a runaway train that catapults the child into the past and face-to-face with previous traumatic experiences. It is not effective to say to a traumatized child: 'Calm down, you are overreacting.' You might as well say this to a passenger on a plane that is coming for an emergency landing. Who are you to decide what is overreacting? (p.150)

With flight the child cries and alerts caregivers to seek protection. Tantrums and aggressive behaviour can be the strategy of flight for terrorized children. But as children are mostly unable to flee, they commonly resort to dissociation, although some children do abscond.

Freezing is usually seen as the child being oppositional-defiant. It is a conduct disorder when negative, defiant, disobedient or hostile behaviour is shown toward authority figures. Common signs and symptoms are temper tantrums, arguing with adults, actively defying rules, deliberately annoying people, unfairly blaming others for mistakes or misbehaviour, being touchy or easily annoyed, angry, resentful, spiteful or vindictive. The adult response to this can be to threaten and demand, which then increases the child's fear.

We have referred above to the interplay between body and mind in understanding human reactions, and mention here of freezing and other symptoms induced by trauma takes us to the somatic aspects of trauma as seen in the theories of van der Kolk, McFarlane and Weisaeth (1996).

Traditional psychotherapy, van der Kolk says, pays scant regard to the post-traumatic bodily experiences. New understandings about the brain show that emotional states originate in our physical condition, for example our body's chemical profile, the state of the internal organs, the contraction of the muscles in our face, throat, trunk and limbs (van der Kolk 2002). The most common and obvious manifestation of this is how we shake and perspire and our breathing rate increases dramatically in stressful situations. According to van der Kolk (2002), these findings should promote awareness, rather than avoidance of somatic states:

> Mindfulness, awareness of one's inner experience is necessary for a person to respond according to what is happening and is needed in the present, rather than reacting to certain somatic sensations as a return of the traumatic past. Such awareness will free people to introduce new options to solve problems and not merely to react reflexively. (p.50)

For van der Kolk, part of the work with those who are traumatized is to help them regain bodily control by reworking the trauma and completing the action. In an interview with Pointon (2004), he says:

> It's via the awareness of deep bodily experience that people can begin to move around the way that they feel – not by keeping it out there. The story of what happened is worth telling, but to change your reaction to it, you have to go via the deep internal felt sense.

The trauma bond

If people know anything about the trauma bond it is usually because they remember the classic case, although not associated with the abuse we are talking about, of Patty Hearst, heir to the publishing company founded by her grandfather, William Randolph Hearst. A group calling itself the Symbionese Liberation Army kidnapped her and she ended up as one of 'them', taking part, apparently uncoerced, in bank robberies. This identification with her captors became so extreme that it was symbolized in her being renamed Tania. Occasionally, other stories come to light whereby bonds are formed between others who have been kidnapped and their abductors. The kidnapper–abductee bond is commonly known as the 'Stockholm syndrome'.

Thus, trauma can be deceptive and have the semblance of a secure attachment within a family. But the trauma bond and secure attachment differ in that attachment is based on love and the trauma bond is based on fear and distorts the child's perceptions. She lives in a state of underlying uncertainty, dependency and apprehension, and so seeks to appease the abuser, to meet, even anticipate, his needs and demands. Children affected by the trauma bond exhibit behaviour that is geared to meeting the needs of the adult or what they perceive those needs are.

This can shape how the child (even when she becomes an adult) conducts relationships, suggesting that they are best lived out in servility and dependence. As she grows up, the child can develop a victim mentality, can become attracted to and invite relationships with powerful people who cause harm and help to reinforce their view of relationships. For adults, the trauma bond can influence how they see themselves as parents.

Ziegler (2002) writes of the trauma bond:

It may seem strange to say that survival can be promoted in negative ways, but this idea is the reality for many abused children. These children develop negative bonds that promote their survival, which are called loyalty bonds or trauma bonds. If someone holds your life in their hands, they are very relevant and

powerful to you. Pleasing such a person, or at least not dis-
pleasing them, becomes critical. Such an experience can rapidly
change an individual in lasting ways. The rape victim, the
prisoner of war, the hostage, and the abused child all have similar
experiences.

For severely abused children, what is happening to them is not
unusual; indeed it is usual – what else do they have to compare it with?
Thus, even when the situation comes to an end, they may not be able to
feel that the trauma is over. Thus, their loyalty to their abuser may
continue and the bond remains as a response to a life-threatening
situation.

Traumatized children, say Perry and Szalavitz (2006), tend to have
'overactive stress responses', which can make them needy, aggressive
and impulsive. Therefore, time and patience are two of the essential
attributes in working with them. Perry and Szalavitz (2006) go on:

> These children are difficult, they are easy to upset and hard to
> calm, they may overact to the slightest novelty or change and they
> don't know how to think before they act. Before they can make
> any kind of lasting change at all in their behavior, they need to
> feel safe and loved. Unfortunately, however, many of the
> treatment programs and other interventions aimed at them get it
> backwards: they take a punitive approach and hope to lure
> children into good behavior by restoring love and safety only if
> the children first start acting 'better'. While such approaches may
> temporarily threaten children into doing what adults want, they
> can't provide the long-term, internal motivation that will ulti-
> mately help them control themselves better and become more
> loving toward others. (p.244)

Loss and love

Curtis and Owen (unpublished) offer a very good way of understanding the interplay between child and primary carer (most commonly
the mother) and child's emotional behaviour after loss, neglect and
rejection. They ask us to imagine two cups half-filled with water. One

cup represents a child and the other a primary carer and the water is the 'life essence'. The child is naturally inclined to relate and will, therefore, give some of their essence to the adult in the expectation that this will be reciprocated. Then the water levels remain constant and enriched. If the child does not receive from the primary carer, her essence is decreased, and, if she continues to give, soon little of her essence will be left. At some point, the child will realize that if she does not stop giving she will run out of her essence and may, in a sense, die. To protect herself the child will cover the cup to prevent losing the last of herself. Unfortunately, with a cover on the cup she will not receive any essence and will remain in the chaotic state which caused her defensive action.

It is an interesting fact of human beings that a child who has been abused can still feel a sense of loss of the person who was the abuser. Many abused children love parents who have abused them and what they want is the abuse to stop. But their separation from the abusive parent, when they go into care or when the parent is sent to prison, is for them a significant loss. Thus, how our sense of self is formed and the effect on it of loss, separation and abuse is a very complicated and delicate process.

CHAPTER 4

Bringing it All Together

Today much emphasis is placed on professionals working together – within agencies as much as between them – although, as repeated reports of inquiries into the non-accidental death of children show, this can sometimes be more the exception than the rule. Yet it is the most obviously necessary of practice imperatives. An adult or a child is a whole person and whilst different professionals bring their own insights and skills to bear in the helping process, a child or an adult can never be treated in isolation from their wider context.

An integrated approach

Before we look at the implications of integrated working for assessment, it is necessary to describe the three elements which make up the recovery team. Key to the SACCS' integrated model are: safety (in place of fear); containment (in place of disintegration); and attachment (in place of detachment). Thus, the model is based on openness, not secrecy; on communication, not avoidance; and on predictability, not inconsistency.

Therapy

Therapy is perhaps the best-known but the most commonly misunderstood aspect of the three elements which make up the integrated model (Rymaszewska and Philpot 2006).

The therapist, working in the space between the inner and outer world of the child as unconscious images emerge in symbolic form, builds a relationship with the child where she can begin to explore that inner world – making use, for example, of techniques like play, music, art, dance and drama – and slowly examine some of the harmful experiences of her past. It is the task of the therapist to help the child unravel her confused and overwhelming feelings, to contain her as she does so and to help her to externalize those feelings so that they cease to have power over her.

The therapist helps the child to reprocess her experiences by addressing the distortions in her thinking, so that the past can fall into perspective. Life-story work informs that understanding of past experiences and people and therapeutic parenting (*see below*) forms the secure base upon which the therapeutic healing can take place.

Therapy is often associated with the idea of client–therapist confidentiality, and this is entirely appropriate in the most common forms of therapy whereby the patient or client attends the therapist's consulting room for a certain amount of time each week or each month. However, given the context of this book, it should be pointed out that in a residential setting therapy is one of the elements of the overall therapeutic provision, and this means that, unlike in a clinical outpatient setting, therapists cannot practise with the same degree of privacy or confidentiality, or, rather, that confidentiality takes a different form. This is because all members of the recovery team – those involved in life-story work and therapeutic parenting – need to know what is happening in the therapy session and how a child is behaving and reacting. Similarly, therapeutic parents and life-story workers share information with their therapist colleagues. Thus, the whole team shares confidentiality (*see below*).

We make various references to all three parts of the recovery team in this book but it should be remembered that they are working hand in hand, each sharing knowledge about the child, even when the child is, at certain times, in the care of different members of the team: the life-story worker, the therapist, the therapeutic parent. This means that a child who is undergoing therapy will, at the same time, be experiencing therapeutic parenting and undertaking the journey that is life-story work.

Life-story work

Although life story work with children who are to be adopted is well established in social work (Ryan and Walker 2003) and there is some work of this kind carried out with older people (Gibson 2004; Haight 1998), the life-story work referred to here is richer, deeper, more detailed and takes considerably more time. It involves the child in both gathering some of the evidence, telling her story, selecting materials to illustrate that story and writing or helping to write the story itself (Rose and Philpot 2005).

Life-story work seeks to answer not only the questions of what, why and when about the child's life, but also whom? Who helped the child or who harmed her? Only when children have the answers can they express how they feel about what has happened to them. Although Connor *et al.* (1985) were talking about life-story work and adoption, their description of what the life-story is about fits well with what we are describing here. It is, they say, about 'unravelling confusion and discarding some of the negative emotional baggage which the child has carried for so long'.

Life-story work attaches importance to the past. However, the past is seen as part of the therapeutic process, as something much more than merely chronological or even factual. As Rose and Philpot (2005) say, 'Life story work is about the people in the child's life, what happened to the child and the reasons why those things happened. It is not, and cannot be a simple narrative or description.' (p.16).

The work requires interviewing people who have been part of the child's life, from family to foster carers, social workers to parents, residential workers to teachers. It involves reading social work and court reports, searching out official documents like birth, marriage and death certificates, and electoral registers, visiting (sometimes with the child) places where she has lived or which are significant, talking with the child at great length and liaising with her current carers (therapist, foster parents and residential workers) and drawing up both family trees and ecocharts as well as helping the child create her life-story book.

Life-story work is based on the belief that none of us can ignore what has happened in the past and then just move on. This is even more so with traumatized children, for to ignore their past and try to move on would be impossible because the past would then always overshadow their present. The past must be faced, understood and, finally, accepted. Then progress – recovery – is possible.

Therapeutic parenting

The third and equally important part of the integrated model is therapeutic parenting (Pughe and Philpot 2007). Children whose abuse and neglect has been so severe will have attachment problems because of interference with their emotional development and their negative experiences. Part of the response to this is to compensate for deficiencies in their parenting with a therapeutic regimen that is accepting and containing. They are being 're-parented' because the structured help that they require gives as near as possible an approximation to the kind of positive parenting which they should have received. Therapeutic parenting is not only about the creation of a physical environment reminiscent of an ordinary home but is also the kind of care, in large and small everyday things, that the 'good enough' parent would have given to the child. It is the team of carers who work in the home who carry out the task of therapeutic parenting.

The majority of children who have been abused will not have received the emotional and physical nurture that is necessary for their development. This early privation or deprivation has left them with critical gaps in their emotional development; they may be left emotionally frozen or fragmented, and have an internal working model which severely impairs their ability to form healthy attachments.

Therapeutic parenting aims to provide a child with an experience of parenting that offers symbolic and actual experiences which seek to fill the gaps in her development. In time this provision will challenge the child's inner working model and enable her to begin to feel differently about herself, other people and the world around her.

An essential part of this work is the opportunity for a child to develop a primary attachment with one person, her key carer. It is through this primary attachment that a child will be able to experience a level of preoccupation, akin to maternal preoccupation normally associated with infancy, through which her recovery can take place. A key carer supported by the recovery team will ensure that all a child's physical, emotional and therapeutic needs are met.

The environment where the child now lives is in itself a therapeutic opportunity and one that that is psychologically, as well as physically significant. Every part of a child's life is seen as having therapeutic potential and, therefore, the home is structured with great attention to everyday details to reflect this.

For children who may have been deprived of so much, emotionally and physically, the home should have a sense of plenty being available: toys, games, art, ornaments, plants, furnishings, comics and books. The home should be child-centred and reflect the personalities and needs of the children who live there. The children live in small family-based homes for up to five children and a care team of ten, giving the children the opportunity to develop relationships within a protected environment.

Through internalizing their attachments and the experiences that children undergo in an accepting environment with therapeutic parenting, they are able to reach a level of recovery which enables them to move successfully on to family placement and achieve their potential.

Confidentiality and professional boundaries

Confidentiality is important in work with children but we have referred above to how the confidential relationship with the therapist takes a different form with integrated working; similarly confidential relationships with all professionals. Confidentiality is shared but this poses questions about professional boundaries. Each professional brings to the child his own particular skills and ways of working. When we understand that the child is seen holistically, then we understand, too, that these skills, perspectives and ways of working are equally important. It is bringing them together in an integrated way rather than practising them separately and in isolation that moves the child towards recovery. Because information is shared when confidentiality is jointly held, then professionals must respect each other's expertise and insights and to be clear about boundaries (Cant 2002, p.270).

Cant (2002) talks of the need to be 'constantly vigilant' about boundaries. She gives an example from her own practice:

> the children inevitably see me about the house at times other than their therapy sessions, but I make it clear that I am 'passing through', and do not get involved in conversations with them, or with other staff, in their presence. If I am inadvertently present during an incident, I will absent myself immediately, and if a child approaches me for assistance, my response is always to refer them to the appropriate adult on duty. Thus the children come quickly to realize that there are boundaries and delineations of role. (p.279)

So, while confidentiality about the child is held within the recovery team as a whole, it is very important that professional boundaries are clear so that there is no confusion between the different areas of work for the child. One way of ensuring this is for the child's therapist and life-story worker always to be different people and for them not to work in the house where the child lives. Therapy sessions should take place at a central location or at least at somewhere which is physically separate from any of the homes where the children live. Similarly with life-story sessions. This allows the child to know that there is distinctiveness and separation between therapeutic parenting, life-story work and therapy, but also that they all communicate and work closely together across their boundaries and share information in her interests. This will be, literally, obvious to the child when there is a handover between therapist and residential care worker. She will also know the whole recovery team is involved in meetings where they consider her.

Integrated working and assessment

It is often the case, even within multi-professional and multi-agency teams, that there will be a lead professional and so it is all the more important to emphasize that assessment is a shared task for everyone in the team. As Kane (2007) says, 'one person cannot hold the key to meeting all the child's needs' (p.17), whereas Ward (2004) states, 'What matters most...is that the whole team is engaged in the process of assessment and in the process of treatment' (p.9). It should never even be assumed that one person has all the answers. We have previously quoted Dockar-Drysdale (1993) as being very explicit when she says, 'all needs assessments must, in my view, be made by a group, *never* by an individual collecting information or depending on interview procedure' (p.94). Indeed, elsewhere Dockar-Drysdale (1990) describes the importance of the whole team working together to understand the child, and even how their own difficulties can affect the child:

> As the unit teams became accustomed to using needs assessment, there was a considerable opening up of communication, especially because, for the first time, people began to take some share of the responsibility for boys' acting out. I felt it was safe to say – and say again – that all acting out results from a breakdown in communication. (p.154)

Integrated working contains a large number of key aspects that underpin the assessment process. Perhaps the most obvious of these is that lines of communication between all the recovery team are always open and clearly defined. Communications should flow between the therapeutic parenting team, the therapist and life-story workers. In addition, all members of the child's recovery team should appraise, update and share new insights, strategies or anxieties with the referring authority.

But it is not only those who are directly treating the child who must be involved, but the wider team as well. For example, it is essential that teachers at the child's school should be involved and brought up to date with all significant events, behavioural changes or any issue that the recovery team feels will affect the child's ability to focus and contribute to her school life. Information from the teacher about the child's school day can also be invaluable. For example, how is she progressing in learning and relationships with teachers and other pupils?

The recovery team must meet regularly to discuss each child and to probe and debate facts and beliefs that are held about her. Recovery assessment meetings offer another forum for the combined team to ask questions about the child and develop a shared language and construct a way of working with the child to achieve her maximum potential to recover.

The recovery team must think about the child together in order to understand each child better. They must identify the stage which a child has reached in her emotional development. A child should be held collectively in mind and the impact of her trauma on the six areas of functioning should be considered. As described earlier (*see* Chapter 2) these areas are:

- learning

- physical development

- emotional development

- attachment

- identity

- social and communicative development.

Integrated working provides a team with a means of tracking progress or highlighting areas of major concern if progress unpredictably slips or appears to go backwards. It also identifies blocks and looks to other members of the team to offer fresh insights or suggestions for strategies in order to move the child forwards. Integrated working offers a potentially creative space for any member of the recovery team to air and reflect upon feelings that the child evokes in them.

The child's internal working model (*see* Chapter 3) should be analysed and a working hypothesis made of what impact it may have on how a child views herself as well as her relationship with the world around her. Strategies, beliefs and interventions should be evaluated, and a consensus needs to be reached about what works and what does not.

Assessment meetings at SACCS are held every six months, chaired by an independent senior practitioner. The team will learn a great deal through the exploration of the feelings evoked in them through being with the child as those feelings can be a projection of what the child herself is feeling and, therefore, if reflected upon can teach us much about the child at that point (*see* Chapter 6). Flynn (1998) refers to 'a culture of inquiry' fostering 'creative and containing work' (p.167).

Multi-systemic therapy

If we talk about each member bringing something different but valuable to work with the child, how do we deal with the many contending therapies, the evidence for which varies? Indeed, the very beginnings of psychotherapy were marked by the secession of first Alfred Adler and then Carl Jung, who had been early followers of Freud. Woods (2003) counsels the creative use of different approaches. For example, a child may be engaged in family therapy whilst receiving individual therapy. Deriving from Pithers and colleagues (1998), Woods (2003) says that 'there should no longer be any need to defend one school of thought against another'. However, he favours the idea, which seems logical in view of this argument, that 'whilst there is little evidence that any one treatment is more effective than another, multi-systemic therapy is…a way of addressing the social, educational, behavioural, and psychological aspects of a young person' (p.29).

Young people who have been abused have various needs which, says Woods (2003), means that 'professional partisanship' must be put aside because of the need to assist them by the most effective means. Crittenden (1997) refers to this as a 'purposefully integrated form of eclecticism' (p.25). Support for this comes from Pithers and colleagues who found that multi-systemic therapy was supported by empirical evidence (p.356). Woods (2003) makes the same point but relates it more generally to our human condition when he says that it 'may well be that a group of theories rather than a monolithic entity provides a more accurate view of complex psychological and social reality' (p.28), adding:

> As a flexible and individualized approach to a wide range of problems MST is proving to be a very significant and non-partisan way forward with psychosocial problems of the more severe kind. (p.29)

Joined-up psychotherapy

Related to this idea of multi-systemic therapy is what Cant (2002) calls 'joined-up psychotherapy, where the insights from individual psycho-therapy are shared with the rest of the staff team in the service of a more profound understanding of the child's internal world'. Equally, this also works the other way, so that the insights of teachers and resi-dential care staff can inform the understanding of psychotherapists. In suggesting this, Cant (2002) introduces a different understanding of confidentiality, which we have advocated: that it is held, not by one individual but the team, 'not in isolated pockets within the community' (p.272).

However, Cant (2002) goes on to say:

> But I also wonder whether there is something more: that, for children of this age, who have already suffered the most appalling degree of deprivation and emotional damage to warrant them being placed in a residential setting, the opportunity for indi-vidual psychotherapy, on top of excellent therapeutic primary care, begins to offer the enormous preoccupation that these children need. As we all know, love is not enough, but neither is ordinary 'good enough' maternal preoccupation. These children

need more than that; they need an extraordinary degree of preoccupation, joined up around them in a safe and containing way.
(p.280)

These may be challenging ideas but they should also be commonplace
in work with children and range far beyond psychotherapy. No one
person holds the solution to a child's problems but a team that works
together may do.

CHAPTER 5

Assessment, Needs and Outcomes

It is simplistic to view assessment as only gathering information to decide on a course of action. This disguises a number of essential ingredients. The Department of Health and the Department for Education and Employment (2000) have summed up what the principles of assessment must be. They are:

- centred on the child
- rooted in child development
- ecological
- ensure equality of opportunity
- work with children and families
- build on strengths, as well as identity difficulties
- inter-agency in their approach to assessment and in the provision of services
- a continuing process, rather than a single event
- carried out in parallel with other action and providing services
- based on evidence.

(p.10)

Three government departments (Department of Health, Department for Education and Employment and Home Office 2000) advise that when practitioners undertake an assessment of a child's developmental needs they should:

- identify the development areas to be covered and recorded

- plan how developmental progress is to be measured

- ensure proper account is taken of a child's age and stage of development

- analyse information as the basis of planning future action.

(p.18)

A critical outcome for care planning in adopting these principles is, according to Kane (2007), 'acquiring knowledge about child development, attachment theory, resilience and understanding risk factors' (p.19). Prior and Glaser (2006) talk about 'clinical usefulness', which they explain as:

> a summary of how useful the assessment might be in a clinical setting, based on what has been said about its established reliability and validity, and an assessment of the ease with which it can be administered. (p.88)

Prior and Glaser (2006) go on to say that this assessment of usefulness takes account of the time and resources needed to train and administer the assessment and what comes out of it.

At the beginning there should be a clear sense of what it is hoped assessment will achieve. We need to look at how a specialist assessment fits into a wider context and ensure that the outcomes of the common assessment framework and *Every Child Matters* (HM Treasury 2003) are the boundaries within which the assessment is carried out. Assessments should identity where a child is in her development, measure and evidence progress, enable plans to be worked out within the context of achieving outcomes and provide a clear format for communication about those outcomes. In assessment it is important not only for team members to think together about the child but to think about the child's needs. Too often in the past the child's primary carers will have thought about her needs in relation only to their own.

In the draft consultation on the framework for assessment, the Department of Health and Department for Education and Employment (1999) say that 'good tools cannot substitute for good practice, but good practice and good tools together can achieve excellence' (p.66). What is needed, then, is an intelligent approach, which embraces both knowledge and the ability to use it to best effect. To do this requires good practice – the combination of knowledge, confidence and skills – which comes from regular training and supervision.

The care plan

It is important when collecting information that we are clear what we want and why we want it, in order to know how we will use it. This knowledge has to be underpinned by gathering information 'in a manner that promotes, or sustains, a working relationship with the children and their families' (Cox and Bentovim 2000, p.3).

More specifically, as Kane (2007) reminds us:

> the care plan contains…the long-term plan for the child and how permanence is going to be achieved. All children who are looked after should have a care plan, personal education plan and health plan in place. (p.8)

What are the wider elements in that plan? Williams and McCann (2006) suggest:

> The care plan is built upon a holistic assessment which identifies development need, the capacity to meet need (parenting capacity and family and environmental factors) and an evaluation of what has happened to the child (history and chronology). The assessment must be continually updated and feed into revisions of the care plan and the review process.

Care planning, once desired outcomes have been agreed, is not something which stands alone: it can only be implemented when we know what the situation is and what needs to be done. Planning is also not something that is one-off and finite, it is a continuing process which requires constant monitoring to observe its effects and the ability to adjust the plan according to continuing evaluation and any changed or unforeseen circumstances. Essential to this are meetings where the plan is reviewed. This is not something for professionals alone because children and young people need to be involved in this and their views taken into account (*see* Chapter 7).

After the assessment, the recovery team develops a recovery plan. As we have said, everyone involved with the child is part of this process and each *part* of the recovery team compares their own assessment, bringing with them their understanding of the child's needs and their own perspective. The team then agrees the key areas of work for the next six months. When doing this, the chairperson, who should be a senior practitioner, offers an external perspective, helps to clarify points and establishes a consistent approach to the assessment and the subsequent plan (*see* Chapter 6).

Tomlinson (in press) has described how the assessment process helps, as follows.

- **To identify, in terms of outcomes, where a child is in her development,** measure progress and outcomes for children, evidence progress and outcomes consistently, work out plans within the context of achieving outcomes and communicate about outcomes clearly.

- **To think about children together** – this is very important for these children who have had lives where the adults caring for them have not been able to think about them and their needs, or in some cases have only been able to think about the child in terms of meeting the adult's need. So we are providing the child with the experience of being thought about in a positive and caring way.

- **To understand children better** – through the assessment we have a better understanding of the child, which enables us to respond more effectively to her. For the child, the experience of being understood may be new.

- **To develop a shared language and approach,** which is very valuable when working in multi-disciplinary teams.

- **To integrate our work in therapeutic parenting,** therapy and life-story, so that everyone is working together consistently and in a focused way to achieve the same aim.

- **To clarify what we need** to put in place to achieve these outcomes.

- **To evaluate our approaches** of what works and what does not.

(pp.6–7)

Subjectivity, objectivity, qualitative and quantative

However, lest we give the impression that an assessment is a clinical gathering of facts, let us turn now to what we might call its human elements: those assumptions and judgements which go into making it. Assessment has to be rigorous but it can never be wholly objective. The impossibility of this is explained by Dockar-Drysdale (1993):

> In order to make any kind of assessment in regard to a person, information must be collected by other people from other people and then communicated by people to people. This final communication is bound to be influenced by all the current factors operating on the lives of the many people involved – above all, the sense of urgency, because of the 'crisis' climate of which I have already spoken. All the *feelings* of the worried people engulfed in the crisis, are going to be in the assessment and also all the feelings of the workers who are managing the assessment. (p.90)

Dockar-Drysdale (1993) later says:

> There will be feelings evoked by the child's personality in those who are dealing with him at such a moment, and also *his* reaction to the strangers who have come into his life which will affect his behaviour. Given such an emotional climate, it may be difficult to sort out the objective reality. This history presented by the parents may omit much, and distort even more (for example,

the mother of battered [*sic*] babies). The child may present a false picture of himself because he will be under great stress: even his intelligence may be blurred by underfunctioning due to emotional disturbance. (p.91)

Dockar-Drysdale (1990), also quotes Robert Langs who, writing of an analyst and patient, said:

The analyst is continuously scrutinizing his own subjective feelings... He must be aware of his own tendencies to distort and misperceive his vulnerabilities, blind spots and defensive needs in the analytic relationship. (p.32)

The questions of subjectivity and objectivity are closely related to the dynamic of the process, which we will discuss later (*see* Chapter 6).

Those who work with children do not live and work in a carefree bubble: their working lives can be very stressful. A part of this is the strong feelings that can be evoked by the child's personality and behaviour. All children react to others, but children who are emotionally damaged can often exhibit extremely strong and negative (as well as overly familiar positive) reactions toward those with whom they have contact. 'A whirlpool of crisis, full of guilt and anxiety' is how Dockar-Drysdale (1993) described this all too familiar situation. It is this, she goes on to say, which can make practitioners' reporting highly subjective. This itself may be exacerbated by imperfect information which parents offer or a child who may give a false picture of herself. There is, though, no escaping this.

It is this understandable tendency to subjectivity which partly make assessments that are jointly arrived at so necessary. Related to this is the use of quantative and qualitative data. We cannot always rely on research as a guide, although, of course, basing what we do on evidence, where it is available, is vital. The outcome data from research may not exist or, if it does, it may not fit the particular case or its circumstances. According to Ball and colleagues (2004), there are benefits in having a mix of quantative and qualitative data gathered from different sources and perspectives. Scoring guidelines and the role of the chairperson both help to contain the tendency to subjectivity within acceptable limits. Alongside this, the significant amount of data recorded daily about each child also helps to balance subjective feelings with tangible realities, such as school attendance, physical health, number of difficult incidents and positive achievements.

But, anyway, the question should be asked: should assessment even aspire to be purely objective? No, because this would reduce children to no more than ciphers on a scoring chart; it would dehumanize them. An open mind is necessary for assessment. If we looked strictly objectively at a child, it might be, for instance, that she appears to be doing well and making progress. But how do we know this? How do we know that she hasn't driven her problems under the surface and what we see now is only that surface? This means that we have to tolerate doubt and uncertainty; we have to be prepared not only to live with them but to recognize that they may be useful to seeking the true picture. Thompson (2000) talks about the 'notion of uncertainty, of no security and no guarantees' as being important for practice. There is a messiness about dealing with human beings that demands a flexibility which is integral to the idea of working with uncertainty. We may seek evidence for how we work but that should not be taken to mean that there are formulaic solutions to people's problems. Dockar-Drysdale (1993) refers to 'the toleration of doubt' and the need to recognize 'the inadequacy of knowledge'.

In fact, the more certain we are, then, at times, the least helpful this will be. For example, let us say that a child is erecting a façade to hide stress: the more that we praise her for showing that façade (or, rather, for the 'good' qualities that that façade shows), the more we are removed from the actual reality of her stress and the reasons for it. If we continue like that, when the stress does emerge it may do so in a shocking and possibly damaging way.

Whatever an assessment tells us, we must retain a healthy scepticism: there are children who will surprise us by not conforming to what we expect and that surprise may be negative or positive.

Common sense and labelling

There are, however, two kinds of subjectivity that need to be guarded against. The first is common sense in the sense of received opinion which is not based on any evidence. Thompson (2000) says that 'common sense' protects dominant ideological perspectives and can deter critical thinking, which, he says raises questions rather than provides answers. In eschewing common sense, he advises, a critical perspective is one which relies on thought rather than 'thoughtless assumption' (p.97).

The second result of subjectivity that can have no place in assessment is labelling a child. Labelling obstructs assessment by failing to see the child as she is. This is sometimes the case but Clough, Bullock and Ward (2006) say that an assessment should be 'used as the basis of a positive plan for [children's] care and treatment rather than as a (possibly unhelpful) label' (p.101). Harvey (2006) says of the educator George Lyward that he was 'passionately opposed to any labelling of a girl or a boy. He regarded labels as masks, and as ways to bind people in' (p.122). Lyward (1958) himself wrote of labels:

> Labels put you in your place, but the place they put you in is on the periphery. The prodding question is a kind of label, a kind of fixative. Not long ago a visiting doctor said to one of our older boys: 'How long have you been here?' The boy replied, looking him straight in the face: 'How long have you been qualified?' (p.8)

A label disguises the child; it doesn't tell us who she really is, it prevents us from seeing that whole self. Dockar-Drysdale (1993) remembered an army psychiatrist who, in a report on a seven-year-old boy who had caused a lot of trouble, described him as 'a potential psychopath'. She wondered about the possible effect of such an assessment on the rest of the boy's life (p.89).

Labels on children, in particular, have a dreadful adhesive capacity: once applied they are very difficult to remove and no matter what happens to the child as she goes through, say, school or the care system that label too easily stays with her, so she becomes not only known by it but it shapes how people react to her almost as if a label had been literally affixed to her forehead.

But the most fundamental kind of labelling is that which the holistic approach avoids. This is where we see the child as her problem or as the sum of her problems rather than as a child first and foremost. It doesn't let us see Lucy, only the self-harmer; it doesn't picture Tom but only the sexually aggressive 10-year-old. It is also a kind of labelling which focuses on the child's deficits rather than her strengths, that sees her as passive, rather than someone who, with help, can participate in her own recovery.

Each with his own

Involving all the team in the assessment means that each person's subjectivity meets with another's to reach a truer understanding of the child. Dockar-Drysdale (1990) talks about the 'context profile' where each child is studied for a week by all members of the household (the residential unit), each recording in detail their experience with a child. She explains:

> We do not admit detached observations into this kind of study, for we need each person's total response to the child, which will be both objective and subjective together. Winnicott once described this by saying in conversation that 'for a moment we see the whole child, with all the bits brought together'. (p.189)

We can make use of objectivity and subjectivity to bring all these 'bits' of the child together. A child's experiences are inevitably subjective and what she feels about an event is more important than analysing the event itself. What the practitioner does is to bring his perspective to bear on that subjective experience, and by sharing that with colleagues comes to an understanding of the experience of the child which is then fed into the assessment. We referred above to Dockar-Drysdale's point (1993) about 'the toleration of doubt'. She recognizes that knowledge is finite and writes:

> I am only urging that we should support each other in the tolera-
> tion of doubt, and recognize the inadequacy of the knowledge on
> which we must depend in order to take action which will affect
> the future life of the person concerned to an extent which we are
> in no position to calculate. (p.92)

Information-gathering is important because it can marshal the hard
facts and offer objectivity when it is due but the assessment process has
also to reckon and make use of those intangibles which can only be
teased out, analysed and discarded or used through a process where
everyone comes together recognizing or being helped to recognize,
their own assumptions and personal perspectives. The life-story
worker provides the whole team with a synopsis of the child's history
and that of her parents and significant family members.

The gift of time

Patience and time are the two most precious gifts that can be offered to
any child but this is even more true for one who is emotionally
damaged. For her, time is the vehicle in which she moves towards
recovery and patience is a means of helping that vehicle to move.

Prickett (1974) talks about this when he describes the regimen
which George Lyward instituted at Finchden Manor, an extraordi-
narily successful educational and therapeutic community, near
Tenterden in Kent, with which Lyward was associated from 1930 to
1973. Prickett (1974) writes:

> So the boys got up each day knowing that there was, among
> other things, time for dawdling, time just to be, and time enough
> for conversational exploring, and so for the gaining of
> knowledge about oneself and others. Such gains and insights
> made the world seem a little less hostile, even manageable. There
> was time for just being – for freewheeling. One boy, when asked
> what the boys did all day, replied: 'I don't know what we do, but
> it's a fine place to be in.' (p.56)

In fact, Harvey (2006) calls Finchden Manor 'a way of life'. The means by which recovery takes place is, of course, complex, highly skilled and fraught with dangers, disappointments and dilemmas. Time *in itself* is not the complete answer. But what space and time, allied with support and patience, offer is the opportunity for the child to be away from the environment which damaged her, a chance to move away from (literal) nightmares and all those things which she believes threaten her, and the assurance that she is safe. In such a physical and emotional environment, where the gift of time is the practitioner saying, 'You are important and worth all this time and effort,' the child can recover her self-esteem, begin to understand that she is lovable and deserving of respect and begin to trust others.

How children will come to see this is shown when Harvey (2006) refers to the fact that 'our unshakable belief that he or she can succeed one day will be passed on to the child, who will realize that we are waiting with and for him and there is time enough for success to come' (p.84).

Writing half a century later and drawing on the latest research, including neurobiology, Perry and Szalavitz (2006) argue that one of the greatest lessons learnt is that of:

> Simply taking the time, before doing anything else, to pay attention and listen. Because of the mirroring neurobiology of our brains, one of the best ways to help someone else become calm and centred is to be calm and centred yourself – and then just pay attention.
>
> When you approach a child from this perspective, the response you get is far different from when you simply assume you know what is going on and how to fix it. (p.244)

To illustrate the importance of time in work with traumatized children, we shall say something about a boy called Tony. He was 11 years old when he was placed in a residential children's home providing a therapeutic service. He had been hugely neglected and deprived throughout his early childhood and both his parents had been severely inadequate in their care of him.

During his first few months in the home Tony was very withdrawn, not particularly demanding, but seemed to be living in a shell unable to show any sign of enjoyment in anything. This continued for over a year and a half with occasional glimmers of humour from him that suggested he was thawing emotionally. However, he was keen not to accept any kind of provision and accepted care as a routine, rather than something that might be special. With the support of the team, Tony's key carer was continually looking for the right moment or opportunity to find a way in.

After about two years Tony asked if he could have a special time with his key carer where he could choose a special food for himself. Following the introduction of this, which he went on to enjoy, Tony explained that when he visited the home for the first time, he could tell it might be a good place because children were allowed to ask for food or take a biscuit. But even though he then saw this every day and was offered the opportunity himself, he was unable to take it as he was terrified of being told off and called greedy. He said that this is what his parents continually had said to him, so not only did he learn never to ask for anything, but he always felt that he was bad for wanting something. From this small example, it is possible to see how many times and for how long something may need to be experienced before any deep change may take place.

But time, in its usual sense, is not only what we give to the child, it is also the minute detail required in assessment. Dockar-Drysdale (1990) tells how she added 24-hour programmes to the needs assessment, which meant that the whole team went over the needs of the child during 24 hours – how she needed to wake in the morning, what happened with regard to her washing and dressing, breakfast time and so on – until they looked at how she went to bed and the needs which surrounded that (Did someone sit with her while she went to sleep? Was there a bedtime story? Was a nightlight on? Was the door left ajar?). Such meticulousness caused the team to think even more about the child's needs and to understand what they were. Had that not been a shared exercise, had each person not told Dockar-Drysdale what their perceptions were of the child's needs, the exercise would not have been a mite as effective as it was when everyone was involved together. As she says, 'A programme like this ensured that a unit team would all know a boy's needs at that time' (p.156).

This emphasizes, too, what we have already said (*see* Chapter 4): that therapy is not something set apart from children's daily lives because their lives are not compartmentalized. Everything – from waking up in the morning to going to bed at night – has an impact on a child. In one sense the whole team are therapists but, importantly, the environment is a healing and therapeutic one and all activity is geared towards the child's recovery.

A means of gauging a child's progress

Vygotsky's (1978) 'zone of proximal development' is a concept which has proven to be influential in education – and particularly in understanding of literacy – and in understanding human development. In a much-quoted passage, he himself described it as:

> the distance between the actual developmental level as determined by independent problem solving and the level of potential development as determined through problem solving under adult guidance or in collaboration with more capable peers. (p.86)

It is the space between the child's current or actual development (emotionally or in terms of learning) and her potential ability or development; the gap between what *is* and what *could be* with the help and support of others. This support is what Vygotsky calls 'scaffolding'. To erect this scaffolding, Vygotsky believed that teachers had to be able to observe acutely the child and where she had reached in terms of learning and what were her capabilities, allowing for her individual needs and their social context. The parallels here with assessment (indeed, with working with children generally) outside of education are obvious.

Vygotsky's ideas are based on the belief that while a child can learn through her own exploration, her development also very much rests on her interaction with others, the help and support that they can offer her and the ability to solve problems together. Development, for Vygotsky, is something which is mediated through things like words, signs and symbols and so on, acquired as the child grows, and these change from being external social phenomena to become internalized (a word Vygotsky uses) as psychological instruments that can be employed independently by individuals.

There are very obvious parallels here with working with children whose development has been arrested through abuse and neglect and also in measuring what we want to achieve through life-story, therapy and therapeutic parenting. But, first, it has to be said, as Aldgate and colleagues (2006) point out:

> If the people around the child are preoccupied with their own cir-
> cumstances, are not interested in the child or have no energy, then
> the child is left to work much more out alone. The neglected
> child's cognitive abilities will gradually develop, but he or she
> will not experience the fun of learning in a social context and the
> learning experiences will not be so rich. (p.188)

Toynbee (2004) reports a study in the USA by Hart and Risley (2002), which found that by the age of four a professional's child will have 50 million words addressed to her, a working class child 30 million and a child where the family is on welfare, only 12 million words. The research went on to analyse the quality of what was being said to the child: the professionals' child received 700,000 'encouragements', the working class child 80,000 and the welfare child 60,000. The language skills of these children at three tallied remarkably with predicted accomplishments at the age of ten. However, the authors found that if very young children were given extensive interaction with teachers this could make up for what they lacked at home.

One assumes that this research was carried out among a general population of children in the three groups (although some of these children are likely to have been abused and neglected). That being so, it is a caution for those who work with traumatized children where the alertness of the practitioner, his preoccupation with the child and his emotional, mental and spiritual energy for the task are every bit as essential as his professional insight and abilities. Without them children's growth to recovery will be slower and less consistent. It also underpins, in this context, Toynbee's point that class (or, in our case, abuse and neglect) need not be a determinate of a child's life chances: intervention works.

Using the zone of proximal development with traumatized children

A most creative practical application of Vygotsky's theory is through the use of the spider diagram, which SACCS has developed. This is a visually striking way of allowing a snapshot of a child's development both at an exact time and over time. In developing this idea, the spider diagram was by far the most popular form of visual representation. This is partly because it captures symbolically the sense of the healthy child and the small or damaged child within. This could be seen as the small 'ego core' of the child as it grows over time toward the 'well-rounded' child. In Figure 5.1 the circumference represents where a child with 'normal' or healthy development could be, and the inner

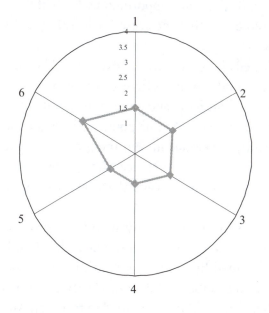

1 = Learning

2 = Physical Development

3 = Emotional Development

4 = Attachment

5 = Identity

6 = Social & Communicative Development

Figure 5.1 *The spider diagram*

shape shows where the gaps are for the assessed child and how far there is to go.

Each part of the recovery team – life-story worker, therapist and therapeutic parents – assesses the child in terms of where she is with regard to the six developmental outcomes: learning, physical development, emotional development, attachment, identity and social and communicative development. They do this by scoring each outcome on a scale of four, with half-scores (e.g., 1, 1.5, 2, 2.5 and so on) allowed. A score of one equates with severe difficulties, whereas a score of four equates with healthy, age-appropriate functioning. The child's development in the six areas may be quite variable. However, to avoid the scoring being too subjective, guidelines help team members. For example, recovery with regard to learning, which is seen as both social and academic, is defined as the child being able to process new experiences and information and hold on to these experiences and to make appropriate choices by using what has been learnt. There are then four sub-sections for each outcome, and for learning they are: understanding cause and effect, taking responsibility for herself, academic progress and the ability to make opportunities. Each of these is explained and each is scored so that the score for learning is the average of the four scores.

The scores are then plotted along the axis and over time. The lines on the graph show both the child's progress for each of the outcomes but also how they come to converge more and more to the point where they reach towards the circumference. At this point we have a child who has a 'normal' or healthy development. But the greater the gap between the inner shape and the circumference, the greater is the child's need for therapeutic support or, as Vygotsky would have said, 'scaffolding'.

The spider diagram allows focus and analysis in order to produce new strategies for the team's work or for it to continue if the child is making progress. Drift is avoided by plotting a child's progress like this, as well as helping all team members think more clearly. It is also a method of finding out where the child is on her road to recovery. Any new behaviours or new information which has come to light recently may be communicated and woven into the proposed strategy of interventions. The recovery team should be encouraged at the meetings to say what they feel about the child and how they view her.

The recovery team should be able to talk about their struggle to absorb the bombardment of powerful projections they receive from the child and how they interpret their counter-transference. Matters such as envy or resentment between team roles may be aired. Feelings of being attacked, either mentally or physically, can be shared with the group and members' support sought if they are experiencing feelings of exhaustion or ambivalence.

The six-monthly meeting, then, offers an opportunity for the team to consider their work together, with the support of the chairperson, so that there is an increased understanding of the child. These processes allow the whole team to assess what is happening to the child and the impact which they, collectively and individually, are having upon her and what stage the treatment has reached: Is it at the end? Does it need modifying? Is it alright for it to continue as it is? Continuing assessment will clarify the answers to these questions and what should happen next.

Each assessment is followed by developing the individual recovery plan. This identifies key aspects of a child's daily living, relationships and engagement in therapy and life-story which warrant individual and more intensive focus and intervention. The assessment thus informs and is realized in the recovery plan. Both assessments and the plans emerge by the team allowing the child's needs to be identified, monitored and met consistently and systematically at her own pace.

Alvarez (1992) reminds us that 'recovery can be a long, slow process, particularly for the children who have been abused chronically at a young age' (p.151). Working with traumatized children is both complex and time-consuming and needs to be underwritten by the utmost sensitivity. The spider diagram, aided by Vygotsky's insights, allows the team to plot progress and ensure a consistency in their approach to the child as she makes that journey towards recovery.

CHAPTER 6

To and Fro
The Dynamic Process

A child-centred approach must mean literally that – in planning a service for a child, in providing treatment, she and her needs are held in mind to the exclusion of all other matters. It is the child's needs which count exclusively during the assessment (and treatment) and that assessment has to be seen from her perspective, and, indeed, is informed by her views (*see* Chapter 7).

It is worth reiterating this because children are not isolated: they live in families or, at very least, they have come from a family from which they may now be separated. Those families may include a mother and a father, but certainly one parent, and they may well have brothers and sisters, as well as other relatives, such as grandparents, who may be near to the child. It is quite possible, indeed highly likely, that these other individuals will also have needs that will be revealed during the course of the child's assessment. There may be problems within the family which also come to light: these may be housing, violence, conflict, separation, mental ill health, disability or substance and alcohol abuse, and, frequently, a combination of several of these. But if those assessing the child pay too much cognizance to these problems (other than any bearing they may have on the child) then the child's needs may well be lost and not identified or, at least, imperfectly identified, in the assessment.

By way of analogy, let us remember that when a mother is caring for her new born baby, she has her in mind even if she is doing something else; for example, she may be carrying out some household chore and her baby may be asleep in another room, but she is ever alert to the child's noises and movement.

Keeping children in mind, then, must be lived out in practice so that, for example, the team must meet regularly to discuss each child and to look at the facts and beliefs that are held about her. Recovery assessment meetings offer another forum for the combined team to ask questions about the child and develop a common understanding about her and construct a way of working with her to help her achieve her maximum potential for recovery.

The team must think about each child together in order to understand her. They must identify where a child has reached in her emotional development. A child should be held collectively in mind and the impact of her trauma on the six areas of functioning outlined earlier (*see* Chapter 2 and Chapter 4) should be considered.

Holding the child in mind is what Cant (2002) terms 'a more total therapeutic experience' of which therapy itself, as we have explained earlier, is only a part (*see* chapter 4). She writes of:

> how vital it is for the child that all the adults involved in their care talk, think and act with a common understanding and a shared purpose. This means that residential staff must talk to teachers, teachers to psychotherapists, psychotherapists to administrative staff – and in all permutations, if the child is to be held in mind and in body, securely, reliably and consistently. (p.267)

Later, Cant (2002) says:

> The sort of children who find themselves in residential provision need more than individual maternal preoccupation. They need the joint, joined-up preoccupation of all the staff who work with them. They need to feel held by the whole community, and to know that the community is more than the sum of its parts; that it cannot be weakened and split, but that it can withstand attacks and survive, and help them to survive. Only then can they begin

to feel held and contained enough to take the enormous risk of making relationships founded on trust rather than mistrust. (p.278)

In the day-to-day work with children, what may seem trivial, or not otherwise readily comprehensible, easily understandable or explainable can, when the child is held in mind and when confidentiality is shared in an integrated team, have meaning. Cant (2002) explains:

> A seemingly unimportant comment from a child can often, when placed in a wider context, together with other people's information and insights, make sense in a way it could never do when it was only an isolated utterance. (p.268)

This is what Cant (2002) calls 'this attention to detail in its every form' and a 'piecing of things together'. But, as she says, it needs practitioners who are '*really* interested and curious – curious to understand how the child feels inside, and why and how they have come to feel like that'. Such a task is about gathering clues, putting the pieces of the puzzle together and making sense of it (p.268).

Dynamics of the process

Integrated working offers a potentially creative space for any member of the recovery team to air and reflect upon feelings that the child evokes in them. As we have stressed previously, assessment is not a mere gathering of the facts, an entirely objective process (*see* Chapter 5). This is evidenced in particular in the dynamics of the assessment process. The chairperson of the assessment meeting, as enabler, analyst and mediator, is critical to this. When talking about the role of a chairperson of a review meeting Kane (2007) says it is:

> to facilitate open and honest discussion around the child, impact on individuals and the organization, feedback on any tensions or complicated dynamics that may become apparent during the meeting, monitor the individual treatment plan and attend the review in order to provide oversight, consistency and continuity to the treatment and target-setting process. (p.26)

However, the chairperson of an assessment meeting may, at times, need to give direction or suggest ways forwards.

The chairperson will have read all the papers before the meeting. He will be familiar with what everyone thinks. He has the facts before him. However, what the written assessments say and what the dynamics of the meeting reveal may vary greatly or may, at very least, cast the written statements in a very different light. He may very soon come to divine that there is something missing, something unspoken, something avoided. He may have been given a picture of the child but not the real child.

Meetings themselves will differ: they may be solemn or jolly; everyone may have much to say or there may be a lot of reticence and holding back; business may be dispatched efficiently and quickly or it may meander and never seem to get to the point. This may often be to do with the child and the effect which the work with her is having on those present.

The chairperson is able to focus on the dynamics of the meeting itself (e.g., the feelings and interactions between practitioners) and use this to further understanding of the child. On occasions, an observer is used to pay specific attention to the process of the meeting. The person in this role makes no direct contribution, but has the opportunity, when the meeting breaks up after an hour, to give feedback to the chairperson. It seems that this role adds to the emotional containment of the meeting, and insights which may have been missed are often contributed during the interval. One practitioner commented, in an evaluation of the assessment process, that the outcomes from the meeting seemed better when there was an observer. It is possible that the person in this role acts as a container enabling others to think more clearly about the child. This is a method that has been used in other settings, such as family therapy.

It is useful to have a photograph of the child projected at the meeting, a reminder of her (literally) present, so that she is held in mind throughout the discussion. In order to involve the child she should be asked to choose which picture she would like displayed. The picture which the child chooses will give an insight into how she sees herself over time. For example, a child may first choose a picture where she is in the background but later choose one where she is much more prominent. This may suggest a greater sense of self-esteem and assertiveness.

It is worth remembering what Cox and Bentovim (2000) have to say about the crowded palette of information that is brought to assessment but also about how it is to be used:

> Assessment does not take place in a vacuum. Assessments benefit from multiple sources of information. Any one source used alone is likely to give either a limited or an unbalanced view. This applies to all the main approaches: interviewing, observation, and the use of standardized tests and questionnaires. Limitations should be recognized. Contrasting data from different methods and/or sources is vital to develop a deeper and more balanced understanding of the situation. (p.3)

One task of the chairperson will be to try to find out how the group or different members see the child. This can be a way forwards, to develop an understanding of what is happening: Does a certain view mean that attitudes are being polarized? Is the child seeing her view of others (e.g., how she believes men and women react) being confirmed in how team members are acting this out? This last point can often be the case and, therefore, there is a need for team members very consciously to break the cycle.

For example, team members can reflect on the ambivalence that Winnicott (1947) shows a mother can have towards her infant: that she both loves and 'hates' her. He gives several examples of what can provoke this. Among them is one when the baby is suspicious, refuses the mother's good food and makes her doubt herself but then the baby eats well when fed by her aunt. On another occasion after an awful morning with the baby, the mother takes her out and she smiles at a stranger who then remarks how sweet the baby is (p.201).

It is quite possible for team members to hold conflicting or ambivalent views of a child without consciously knowing it; for example, they may speak in the meeting very positively about her but when it comes to scoring may score her very poorly, and the opposite may be true: their high scoring may vary with their expressed opinion of her (for scoring, *see* Chapter 5). Where this ambivalence is denied, this is unhelpful and can be damaging to the child as she is also being denied a real and meaningful picture of herself.

Thus, the facts will be available but there will also be the subjective feelings. Where these are openly expressed and acknowledged they can be helpful, but sometimes they can be hidden by people's ambivalent feelings and reactions and so are unhelpful. It is natural that strong negative feelings for a child or sexualized feelings will be denied but none the less it is necessary that they be brought to the surface.

Let's give an example known to one of the authors (Tomlinson). An assessment meeting was discussing a child whose mother had died giving birth to him. There was an obvious need to work with him because he was feeling responsible for this. However, this very germane fact was being ignored both in the work being done with the child and also in the meeting. One key member of the team said nothing in the meeting and it only emerged, by chance discussion in a break, that this team member was pregnant. And so the terrible experience of the child and the tragedy of his mother were directly affecting her own reaction and feelings because of her pregnancy. The team had then responded in a protective way to the very real anxiety involved and avoided the subject altogether.

Transference and counter-transference can, then, often be at work in these meetings and so the chairperson's role can be useful in helping to express and understand what is happening. Acknowledging feelings of ambivalence within the team can enable a more rounded picture of the child to be reflected back to her.

Transference and counter-transference

Transference is when someone unconsciously directs their feelings for one person onto a third person (or, in the case of the pregnant team member mentioned above, transfers feelings about another to themselves). Children harbour all manner of feelings about those whom they have known – parents, other family members, carers, other staff – and they will often transfer these onto those who currently work with them. These may be positive or negative, sexual and non-sexual.

The response to this transference is called 'counter-transference' and the person working with the child must bear in mind whether the child is trying to recreate in him a figure from her past life and thus guard against any reactive feelings, such as anger, fear, frustration or resentment, on his part because this will serve to reinforce the negative feelings which the child previously felt.

A good description of how counter-transference can work, albeit in a different context to that which we are writing about, is given by Aiyebusi (2004) who explains:

> As professionals, we come to the workplace with our own traumas, losses and vulnerabilities, sometimes processed but sometimes unprocessed. Time and again we find that nurses and healthcare assistants who engage with this population of women [in secure psychiatric services] finding themselves disturbed by their work, occasionally to the point of breakdown. It seems that existing defences are no longer effective. The interaction between patients' unprocessed traumatic experience and that experienced by members of staff can amount to a toxic combination. Physical and psychological sickness is then experienced within the staff group... Processing such toxic emotional material is extremely difficult, given the potency of experience and since the counter-transference includes humiliation, exposure, rage and loss, the risk is that instead of processing, professionals act out within the staff group so interactions occur in hurtful ways, including bullying, aggressive practical joking, gallows humour, gossiping or backbiting. Another way of acting out includes launching envious attacks on colleagues who are getting something good like a course or clinical supervision. (pp.52–53)

Menzies-Lyth (1988) says:

> All staff working with these [emotionally damaged] children need to be able to absorb powerful projections from them, think

about them [together with other staff] and return the projections in a more benign state. This often means tolerating extreme anxieties. (p.269)

Hunter (2001) refers to 'trauma fragments' being 'toxic and powerful'. These, she says, are a professional hazard and she continues:

I say this because such experiences stay with you and sadden and burden the recipient as well as adding to one's understanding. I have learned therefore to be cautious and respectful of my [patient's] reluctance to tell or revisit emotionally traumatic events. These happenings are hard to bear even at second-hand. (p.161)

Working in a team not only helps create a holistic picture of the child, it also allows staff to discuss together how they can each deal with the volley of projection and transference which children give to them and how they interpret their counter-transference. It is important that those negative responses, against which they must guard when aware of the counter-transference, may be talked about openly. In this way, team members become more self-aware and effective in their work with children.

CHAPTER 7

A Time to Listen
Putting the Child at the Centre

It has become axiomatic in social care generally, but in children's services in particular, that what shapes services should be the views of those who use them. Services users' needs are rightly required to predominate above the demands of those who provide services. This can only be done if the process of involving service users is integral to service planning.[7] However, as this is something too often honoured in the breach than the practice, it is all the more worth restating. Such a principle gives dignity, purpose and a degree of control to the service user, but it is also the most efficient way of providing services. As Kane (2007) reminds us, 'research suggests that listening and really involving children and young people is the key to effective care planning'. Timms and Thoburn (2003) say the same thing when they say, 'experience tells us that plans have a better chance of success where the children themselves have been involved in their preparation'. Almost any research looking at the views of vulnerable children and young people, and particularly those who are looked-after, has found that the one thing that they seek is to be listened to and what they most resent is not being listened to. We also know that what children and adults understand by listening differs. For a child it means that something will happen as a result of being heard, whereas for the adult it is more to do with the respect he gives to the child by listening to her.

The present philosophy about the central place of users may be traced in different services, but most particularly for those for people with learning disabilities, with the growth of the self-advocacy movement in the 1980s, but, for adults generally, (Beresford and Croft 1980) and, some way behind, the White Paper, *Caring for People: Community Care in the Next Decade and Beyond* (DoH 1989), and the resulting NHS and Community Care Act 1990 and subsequent guidance (Social Services Inspectorate 1991). For children and young people there was the 'Who Cares?' movement of the 1980s and then the Children Act 1989. The latter states the obligation that:

> (4) Before making any decision with respect to a child whom they are looking after or proposing to look after, an authority shall, so far as is reasonably practicable, ascertain the wishes and feelings of:
>
> the child;
>
> his parents;
>
> any person who is not a parent of his but who has parental responsibility for him; and any other person whose wishes and feelings the authority consider to be relevant.
>
> (5) In making such a decision a local authority shall give due consideration – having regard to his age and understanding, to such wishes and feelings of the children as they have been able to ascertain;
>
> to such wishes and feelings of any person mentioned in subsection (4) (b) to (d) as they have been able to ascertain; and
>
> to the child's religious persuasion, racial origin and cultural and linguistic background.

(Section 22)

Nine years later, the Commons Health Select Committee document, *Second Report of the Health Select Committee – Children Looked After by Local Authorities* (House of Commons 1998), said, 'if children in general are a vulnerable group, children looked after by local authorities are acutely vulnerable. It is all the more important that their voice should be heard by people in positions of authority' (p.xlviii).

However, this is easier said than done. Not only is there the matter of how resource constraints determine what has now come to be called 'choice', but, perhaps more problematically, the belief that listening and involvement are vital has not brought with it any clear agreement on what these mean. Sinclair (1991) has suggested that consultation and choice have to be set within boundaries. We also have to ask whether practitioners and agencies have made that internal change in culture and thinking, that revolution whereby they genuinely respect what children and young people (indeed, service users generally) have to say. We have to ask, too, whether they are willing to act on it where they can, and to accept the challenges to their own ways of working and assumptions that that implies.

As Ball and colleagues (2004) say:

> Culture change is, without doubt, the most difficult and least understood area of organizational life. A new culture is not a thing that can be simply installed, or imposed by managers. So how can we create cultures within and across health and social care agencies that understand their purpose in terms of clear, user-valued outcomes? (p.17)

The first step in answering that question must be a respect for what children have to say arising from their own experience. But even then practitioners and agencies must give support to children and young people to allow them to say what they wish to say; after all, being a child and being vulnerable is a double obstacle to facing what may seem the monolithic structure of 'the system'. Practitioners then have to use methods of communication which children and young people find comfortable and can use and speak a language in which children feel able to communicate. They must ensure that children and young people have to hand the information they need in order to make choices and express themselves. Just as children should be allowed to move at their own pace, so ways and means familiar to them should be used, like making use of practical aids to help them. For example, play people and other toys, play-dough, paper, crayons and so on are things which can both help children express themselves and also allow the practitioner to communicate with the child.

One practical example of how a children's trust has set out its principles and practice is that of the Hertfordshire Children's Trust Partnership's Framework for Involvement, to which Kane (2007, p.30) draws attention. Work which is centred on children and young people, says the Trust, should:

- regard them as experts at this point in their lives

- value the perspective which derives from their own experience

- be ready to listen to them when they are ready to speak, not just when adults require them to do so

- ensure that they feel safe

- use language and methods of communication that are inclusive and engage the child and young person and mean something to them.

The trust goes on to say that children and young people may be empowered by:

- giving them support and access to relevant information

- ensuring that the choices available to them are both real and appropriate

- getting their consent to participate but also giving them the chance to withdraw if they want to

- having agreements about confidentiality

- assisting them in being able to talk with those who take decisions

- ensuring that they have access to a complaints or representation procedure, with mechanisms for informal feedback

- offering support from a trusted or independent person or advocate, who could be someone of their own age group or an adult

- offering accredited training.

Listening implies conversation, the give and take which allows agreement and ways of advance. A baby's first sounds are not always directed to anyone in particular, they are unfocused gurgles. But from the beginning a mother talks to her baby and the baby hears and responds, at first with gurgling and 'nonsense' noises and then slowly forming recognizable sounds that then become refined into words. This is how a baby develops speech. Speech is the most basic and necessary of human skills. So when we listen to the child about the planning of services or about the treatment she will receive, we do not do so in order to say, 'Yes, I agree' or 'No, I don't agree and we will do it my way'. We do it to start a conversation, with the to and fro which that entails and the reaching of common understandings and agreements. However, that said, it is wise to bear in mind what Sinclair (1991) cautions:

> Consulting with a child does not mean that they are responsible for the final decision, nor does it mean letting the child have their own way. For participation to be positive everyone must be clear about what choices are and are not available and why.

For anyone, not to be listened to over the simplest of matters is disempowering; it sets us back and removes a degree of our independence and, *in extremis*, makes us passive and can destroy our self-confidence. For those who have been abused, such treatment is far more serious and emotionally and psychologically far-reaching. Abuse creates an enormous sense of powerlessness: the person or child who has been abused has felt used and unable to stop the abuse and has a sense that no one has protected her from what has happened. She lacks control not only over her own self but over her life. Children who have been traumatized through abuse feel this even more acutely. This is because, as Perry and Szalavitz (2006) say, 'trauma at its core is an experience of utter powerlessness and loss of control, [and] recovery requires that the patient be in charge of key aspects of the therapeutic intervention' (p.245).

Thus, those working with such children need to listen to them, to understand their feelings, perspectives, perceptions and fears, and work at their pace. This is because recovery is about restoring or establishing for the child a sense of self and a sense of control, to allow her to break free of the feeling of helplessness. It is about not compounding or repeating some of the effects of abuse by increasing the sense of power-lessness and lack of control. Through the process of help that is offered to her, the child should feel that she has some control; that she is living her healing. There is no alternative, as Perry and Szalavitz (2006) write:

> Over and over again, the research finds that if you use force, if you push people to open up when they aren't ready, if you require par-ticipation in therapy, if you don't respect individual differences, then your treatment can actually do serious harm. Because safety is critical to recovery and force creates fear, coercive therapies are dangerous and ineffective for victims of trauma. (p.245)

The child and the plan

It will be seen from the above that involving children is vital to the success of any plans being made for them – whether plans for recovery or plans for placement. However, while children must be allowed to make choices and participate at their own pace and to suit their develop-mental age, there are also practical considerations to bear in mind. Involvement may be a 'Good Thing' but if it remains an ideal, without the practical underpinning to make it a reality, it will be only that – no more than a pious aspiration and it will not have any real meaning.

This, of course, raises the question of the extent to which the child's view should prevail, because, as we have said, we need to both define the service user (child? parent? local authority?) and what kind of service is needed and what outcomes are planned for. Tomlinson (in press) suggests that children's views, wishes and preferences should be included as much as possible but that outcomes should ultimately be agreed with the parent, the local authority or both. It is to them, he says, that the service provider is responsible. Tomlinson (in press) quotes Willis (2001), who said: 'Users may feel dissatisfied because the service was imposed on them, even though it might have a beneficial outcome' (p.143). Tomlinson responds that 'the focus on issues of choice for the user, or being involved, should not detract from determining whether the user has actually benefited from the service' (p.6).

Involving children, then, is not so much a dilemma but a matter of negotiation, sound principles and, not least, humility, whereby participation in the process (and this is especially so for children) must be based on a number of factors, not least a child's developmental age. But involving them must also be encouraged as far as is practicable. This will challenge practitioners and agencies to put aside old ways of doing things. It may be as much a new turning, in its way, for the professionals, as it is for the children with whom they work. By giving confidence to the child (which will have positive repercussions outlasting involvement in assessment and planning), practitioners will gain a new confidence in themselves.

Grace

A Child, an Assessment and a Plan[*]

Grace Stephens is 11 years old and her own history shaped her childhood but, at the same time, it is not untypical of that of many children who have been traumatized: shifting relationships within the family, violence towards her and witnessing the violence between her mother and father. And, again, as is so often the case, a disturbed family history is part of her own parents' lives.

Natalie Porter, Grace's mother, was 19 and her father, Grant Stephens, was 20 when she was born and her mother already had another daughter and a son by two different men.

Grant had been cared for by his mother after his father left the family before he was one year old. He described himself as having a difficult childhood and that he didn't have a good relationship with his father. Following the birth of his brother when he was 18 months old, his mother suffered post-natal depression. During his adolescence

---

*   For the purpose of illustration we have focused on the first assessment that took place after 3 months, the third assessment after 15 months and the sixth after 32 months. As space considerations preclude our looking at the whole of each assessment, we have chosen to look at one of the six areas: emotional development. The assessment questions are given together with practitioners' responses. For assessments one and six we also look at how Grace was assessed in relation to her internal working model and her overall development. The spider diagram, which shows how Grace was scored in the complete assessment, including the area of emotional development, is shown at the end of each section.

he became involved in criminal activity and by early adulthood served custodial sentences.

Natalie's mother and father (Grace's grandparents) separated when she was very young and they cared for her, though separated. She says that her childhood was difficult and that there was little attachment between herself and her mother. She was physically assaulted as a child by both her mother and her father, and she has witnessed domestic violence between them.

Natalie and Grant's daughter's life was to have some disturbing echoes of their own upbringing. Theirs was a volatile, immature and violent relationship, which ended shortly after their daughter's birth. Concerns were raised about all three children when Grace was five months old and she was admitted to hospital and recorded as failing to thrive, and an initial case conference was called following concerns about the safety of all the children, who were allegedly physically abused by Grant.

All three children were placed on the child protection register under the category of physical abuse. Shortly after this Natalie and Grant were reunited, though it was not long before violence led to another split. Natalie then showed signs of improved stability and the children were deregistered and the social services department closed the case when Grace was 18 months old. Despite the case being closed concerns continued about non-accidental injuries and sexualized comments made by the children.

When Grace was two her mother moved in with a new partner, Neil, who was only 16 years old. Within a month referrals were made that led to a child protection case conference being called. It was reported that the children were often dressed inappropriately and showed signs of non-accidental injury. A decision was made to place all the children again on the child protection register, this time under the category of neglect. Five months later they were taken off the register again.

During the next year various concerns were again raised about the children's sexualized behaviour and allegations of abuse against Natalie. The children were again re-registered and deregistered.

By the time Grace was four, her mother Natalie, who was still with her new partner, Neil, was struggling to cope with the children, and Grace, her brother and sister, her mother and partner were living with Grace's maternal grandmother. Further evidence of abuse and neglect by Grace's mother and partner transpired. Grace made clear and consistent disclosures against her mother's partner implying that he had sexually abused her, but the subsequent investigations found no clear evidence for prosecution. However, all the children were re-registered – this was for the nineth time – under the category of neglect and sexual abuse.

Grace's grandmother complained to the social services about her difficult behaviour and Grace was placed with foster parents when she was four and half, along with her half-brother and half-sister. The foster parents recalled how Grace arrived with a bin-bag of belongings and that she was very upset and was crying. Grace's mother and partner Neil showed improved stability and a plan was made for her half-brother and half-sister to be returned to live with them but it was deemed that it would be too difficult for them to take Grace as well. Her half-brother and half-sister went back to their mother and her partner, but within six months the rehabilitation broke down.

Grace's foster carers reported that she harmed herself, had tantrums and showed sexualized behaviour. But, when she was five and they could not offer her a long-term placement, Grace was put forward for adoption. Before the planned adoption took place Grace's foster mother died suddenly. After this the placement was fraught with raw emotion which indirectly led to an adoptive family being identified. Introductions to the family broke down owing to Grace's clear view that she did not want to leave her foster father and the potential adopters' realizing that they would not be able to cope with her behaviour. Grace remained with her foster father, who was struggling to cope after his wife's death, but a year later, when Grace was six and a half, the placement broke down because of her increased verbal abuse and uncontrollable behaviour.

During the next six months Grace had six foster placements, lasting one week, two weeks, two days, three months, five days and two weeks, respectively. The reasons given for such rapid turnover were stated as violence towards foster carer's son, which resulted in him having to be admitted to hospital, excessive temper tantrums, verbal aggression, kicking, biting and punching a foster carer, aggressive outbursts coupled with suicidal threats, hurting family pets, and sexualized behaviour.

Grace was admitted to SAACS' Beech House when she was eight, after a three-week plan that incorporated visits and meetings with the adults at Beech House.

First assessment: After three months
Emotional development

Here, we are concerned with the child's capacity to cope with, express and understand emotions, both in themselves and in others. The areas for consideration, along with examples of the questions which allow us to define them, are as follows.

- **Emotional regulation:** Emotional expression (How does she express herself? Do expressions of emotion equate to the emotional experience?) and internal experience of emotions (Does she experience distress? Is emotional distress extreme in relation to its cause? Is she overwhelmed by her emotions?).

- **Disruption of others:** Does she disrupt an activity between others? How does she manage jealousy and attention given to peers?

- **Range of emotions:** Is she able to experience a range of feelings like, sadness, happiness, anger? Does she recognize these feelings in others?

- **Capacity for empathy and sympathy:** Does she feel concern for others and make appropriate reparation? Is she able to take the perspective of another person, to step into their shoes?

- **Guilt:** Does she show a capacity for appreciation of the hurt or disappointment she may have caused? Does she seem to feel appropriate concern for her actions?

- **Choice selection:** How does she consider options and make choices? Does she seem to become overwhelmed by uncertainty?

Questions are responded to separately and the following is a selection of the responses to all of the six questions by practitioners.

Grace mostly uses anger to express herself and this is often extreme in relation to what has happened. She often shows tears through frustration. Grace can be completely overwhelmed by her emotions and her underlying distress is more evident when she comes down from her anger. (*Therapeutic parenting team*)

Grace regularly disrupts an activity between others and this mainly seems to be a result of her jealousy. Besides disruption she manages jealousy and attention given to peers through anger and manipulation. (*Therapeutic parenting team*)

Grace feels 'locked into herself' in the most part. She does not seem to be able to take the perspective of another person. She does not tend to appreciate the hurt or disappointment she may have caused. Grace does not seem to feel appropriate concern for her own actions. Grace can be superficial and fake guilt to have her own ends met. (*Therapist*)

Grace does not seem overwhelmed by choices and will consider options before making a choice. (*Life-story worker*)

Grace lacks emotional regulation – indicating that she still requires a high level of attunement and soothing, etc. from adults. (*Therapist*)

I do not see Grace with others but in therapy she acts out extreme jealousy and feelings of abandonment. (*Therapist*)

Grace has begun to 'own' some responsibility for her actions – however, she easily becomes overwhelmed as she feels she is to blame for things that have happened in the past. (*Life-story worker*)

Overall development

Grace's level of functioning and emotional age, any specific areas of concern, sexual development or concerns:

> She functions as a much younger person than her chronological age. Often, her functioning is toddler-level and can, at times, feel more like a young infant. She can behave at her age-appropriate level but cannot sustain this for long periods. She can be sexually provocative with her body language towards children and adults, which is a concern. Grace tries to completely blank out her emotions in therapy sessions.

The internal working model

Grace's view of herself, others and the world.

> Naughty and bad. Not nice to be around. Ugly and fat.

> They [carers] know too much. They can't be trusted and hurt me.

> I can't trust anyone; people just want to hurt me.

Grace's view of the outside world is that it is unsafe with adults who will hurt children and cannot be trusted. There is no place for her in the outside world.

Scoring the assessment

As discussed earlier (*see* Chapter 5), as well as providing anecdotal statements about the child the assessment process requires that the child's progress is also scored. When assessing a child it is necessary to think about the developmental norms for children of similar ages. The child is scored in comparison to what we would expect of a healthy child of similar age. A score of:

- 4 = positive functioning in this area, with possibly minor concerns
- 3 = moderate concerns, with one or two aspects to address

- 2 = substantial concerns, shows some signs of progress but a range of aspects to address

- 1 = severe concerns, indicates poor functioning in this area.

To ensure consistency in our assessments of children it is important that we maintain a balanced view of the child, keeping specific incidents or aspects of behaviour in perspective alongside the child's overall behaviour. The aim is to clarify the areas where a child needs more help and support in order to progress their recovery. When considering a child's progress we recognize that growth is not always linear. A traumatized child finding containment, warmth, safety and positive caring may need to regress in order to progress. Similarly, a child may take two steps forwards and one back.

To support consistency in assessment, scoring guidelines are provided. Under each of the assessment questions there are four sets of scoring indicators, one for each of the assessment scores. The child is scored against the indicator set that most closely matches the child. This does not mean that the child's behaviour and development will exactly match the indicator, but the one chosen is closest to how the child generally is. For instance, the indicator sets under the emotional development question on 'disruption of others' are, as follows, a score of:

- 1 = Cannot cope with more than one relationship. Needs constant adult support. Very jealous and possessive: will become aggressive if not given instant gratification.

- 2 = Will seek adult attention and is disruptive if cannot get her own way.

- 3 = Is able to function without adult attention; enjoys contact with other children, but becomes argumentative if she feels threatened. Does not resort to violence.

- 4 = Is able to cope with multiple relationships and generally not feel threatened by others.

These indicators spell out what an outcome looks like and provide a sequence of progress towards a child's achievement of positive outcomes. There are four stages of progress identified and moving between them takes considerable time. If it is felt that a child is between two of the scores, half-points may be used. How were Grace's scores plotted on the first spider diagram (Figure A.1)? It should be noted that while the axes are numbered one to six they are neither hierarchical nor sequential in terms of the child's development.

As we can see, everyone sees a child who is extremely damaged in her development and who has huge needs. However, there are differences in the three pictures. We often see this with a child like Grace, a child whom Winnicott (1962) may have called 'unintegrated', or Solomon and George (1999) a child with 'disorganized attachment'. She may be different things to different people at different times, compliant one minute and chaotic the next. As a reaction to her traumatic experiences Grace had developed a protective shell which she presented with a degree of success to the therapist and life-story worker. The therapeutic parenting team with whom Grace lived were exposed to the small and extremely traumatized child inside the protective shell.

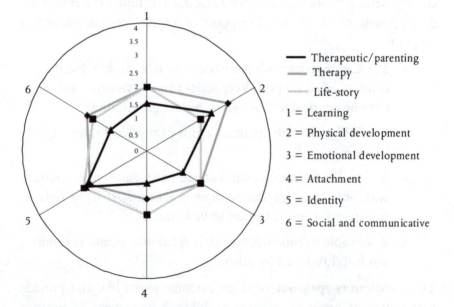

Figure A.1 *Grace's scores on the first spider diagram*

Third assessment: After 15 months

Under the section on emotional development, as explained above, the following observations were made.

> Grace shouts and can be violent when she is expressing emotion but is more able to show sadness and understand this feeling. (*Therapist*)

> Grace will see injustices very quickly if she feels that she is being treated differently or not 'getting' things she would like. She may try to jeopardize outings if she isn't going. She does not manage jealousy well and finds it hard to see Beth happily occupying herself or playing with others, and may try to disrupt this or the atmosphere in the house so that activities are spoilt. (*Therapeutic parenting team*)

> She is highly aware of how everyone is feeling in the house and can sometimes use people's vulnerability to control the situation. Grace can see things from another persons perspective and can show concern if she has not been responsible for causing the upset. (*Therapeutic parenting team*)

> In the aftermath of causing hurt, etc. Grace tries to avoid feelings of guilt, but after a time to reflect she does seem to feel some level concern. However, she may repeat the hurt she has caused to the same or different person and go through the process again. (*Therapeutic parenting team*)

> Grace can be extremely jealous of others. This is a difficult emotional area to cope with due to past deprivation. (*Life-story worker*)

> She is able to experience a wide range of feelings but will actively try to push them aside in an effort to cope. (*Therapist*)

> She has the capacity to be empathic and will show this in therapy. She will often take on the role of being a good mum in role-play. However, in real situations making reparation could pose difficulties. (*Therapist*)

Grace can be sexually provocative. She has said that sexually touching other children is not wrong. She admitted having touched the children and threatened them to stop them telling. This is particularly worrying and needs urgent attention as Grace approaches puberty. (*Life-story worker*)

Grace needs nurture but struggles to accept it and tries to maintain she does not need adults to care for her. There is a sense of abandonment and rage underneath this exterior. (*Therapeutic parenting team*)

Grace is beginning to try and look at others' emotions and will show concerns for others. She will try to hide her guilt from others although she can show concern for others quite openly. (*Therapeutic parenting team*)

Grace needs help to make choices greater than 'yes' or 'no', and can find too many changes overwhelming. (*Life-story worker*)

Let us now look at the spider diagram from this assessment (Figure A.2).

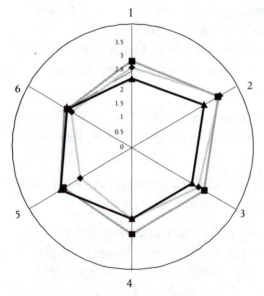

Figure A.2 *Grace's scores after 15 months*

We can see that Grace is filling out in her development and appears to be developing consistently in most areas. The differences in how she is perceived are becoming smaller. Through the integrated work of the recovery team the fragmented aspects of Grace's fragile personality were held together and reflected back to her in a consistent way. This gradually enabled Grace to internalize a more balanced and connected, rather than a fragmented or split, sense of self.

Sixth assessment: After 33 months

Under the section on emotional development, as explained above, the following observations were made.

> Grace is able to access her inner feelings and display empathy towards others. This is often in proportion to the prevailing situation. (*Therapeutic parenting team*)

> Grace finds it difficult to manage two relationships at the same time and will display jealousy when she perceives someone getting more attention than herself. There are occasions when Grace can manage this in an age-appropriate manner. (*Therapeutic parenting team*)

> Grace still tends to cover up emotions with anger as she finds this easier to display. Recently, Grace has learnt to laugh more and can laugh at herself which is a crucial development for her. (*Therapist*)

> Grace has developed the ability, although in its early stages, to show empathy towards others and see things from other people's perspective. Recently, Grace has shown compassion for others and, with help, is able to accept that she is wrong and will attempt to put things right and accept the consequences of her actions. (*Therapeutic parenting team*)

> Grace knows when she is in the wrong and can take responsibility for what she has done. However, if Grace believes that she is in the right, it is difficult to help her to feel any sense of guilt for what she has done. (*Therapist*)

Grace is able to make appropriate choices and is seldom overwhelmed by what is offered. Grace will seek out adult guidance and try to find out as much about something before making a choice. She appears to enjoy the prospect of choice as part of her personal and social learning. Sometimes she will look for guidance or approval, but this is age-appropriate. (*Therapeutic parenting team*)

I rarely see Grace being disruptive of other activities around her and am aware that she is more able to get along with others in her peer group since switching from primary to secondary education. (*Life-story worker*)

Grace has been able to work through and acknowledge a wide range of feelings that she may have encountered in her life. Most of the feelings symbols cause Grace no great worries; however, she always struggles whenever anything sexual is mentioned and when the picture that was chosen for 'sexing' is introduced. (*Life-story worker*)

Grace's overall development

At school Grace behaves in a way that is consistent with her age and development and ability. Grace is a popular child both with adults and peers. However, in the home the situation is different. Grace feels that she does not fit in and reverts to behaviours that make her feel safe and are reminiscent of when she first moved to Beech House. (*Therapeutic parenting team*)

The one concern we do have is in prolonging Grace's stay at Beech House. She is clearly well in advance of her group and has shown a degree of recovery that allows us to feel confident that Grace could achieve well in a family home. (*Therapeutic parenting team*)

Grace's internal working model

She has a more positive image of herself but can still tend to see herself as unlovable and unwanted. In some sense there is a feeling of being the victim. (*Therapeutic parenting team*)

She really likes her carers, although she would have you believe otherwise. Since being at Beech House she has shown that she has a capacity to form relationships based upon mutual understanding and trust that have come through some difficult periods and still remained as important. (*Therapeutic parenting team*)

She alternates between seeing the world as an exciting place to one that is scary and has the ability to hurt her. This seems consistent with her move towards adolescence as well as reflecting her history. (*Life-story worker*)

Let us now look at Grace's next spider diagram (Figure A.3).

We can see that Grace appears to be on the journey to recovery. The zone of proximal development is smaller; she needs less help to

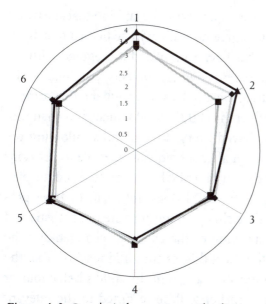

Figure A.3 *Grace's sixth assessment spider diagram*

function to her true potential. There are still areas of difficulty and underlying fragility. We also see Grace's behaviour is more consistent, at different times, with different people in different situations. She is becoming integrated and her attachments are more secure. However, as we have said, recovery is not a cure but a process of evolvement and can be considered a life-long journey. To consolidate Grace's growth she will need a carefully planned transition into a family placement, providing continuity in her care and understanding of her needs. The transition should happen at the child's pace, involving close work between present and new carers.

Individual recovery plan

The individual recovery plan will be completed within the first month of a child's placement, and from then the plan will be used as the basis for work with her. The aims of the individual recovery plan are to describe the child's current behaviour, to state our understanding of her behaviour, to state the aims for achievement in the next six months and to state how we will enable the child to achieve these aims, including timescales where helpful.

The recovery team discuss the plan with the child so that she is able to identify her own aims and agree how she will be helped to achieve them. Once the initial plan has been formulated it is agreed with the child's social worker and parents (where parents continue to be involved). The plan can then be used as a document that can be reviewed and adapted to reflect the child's development and changing needs. The plan is fully reviewed every three months following the initial recovery assessment, then after subsequent assessments. Reasons for adapting the plan could be that the child has progressed and the plan should develop accordingly, the child does not seem to have progressed and the plan should be changed, the aims are not realistic and need adjusting, our understanding of the child has changed and the plan may need to change to reflect this, or the child may ask that the plan be changed. Any significant changes in the child's behaviour or the approach to the work with her will be recorded in the relevant section. This will then give a continuing picture of change and development in each area, showing how outcomes are being achieved.

The child's needs and approach to working with her are considered in relation to all of the following areas: washing and bathing; mealtimes; in-between times; house meetings (where children and adults discuss matters related to daily living); play and activity; travel to and from school; education (academic progress, relationships with children and teachers, support needed throughout the school day); sexual education (at school and home); bedtimes; sleeping; waking up; relationships with adults (staff) and special provision; relationship with children and young people; types of difficult behaviour; risks involved; activity and behaviour outside the home; contact with parents, family, social worker and others; physical health; sexual development/concerns; moving on from SACCS; therapy and life-story.

As with the assessment it is important that there is a holistic approach to the individual recovery plan, with clear links between the different areas. For example, a difficulty or achievement in any one area may have consequences in other areas. An identified gap in one area may be targeted by directly working in that area or more indirectly by interventions in other areas. For instance, if a child is struggling with academic work at school, more support with homework, encouragement and praise may help. On the other hand, the difficulty may be related to an anxiety about other children, separation from home or a physical problem, such as enuresis. In support of this way of thinking, Clifford-Poston (2001) asks the question: what does a child need in order to learn? Her answer is 'a secure base from which to venture out into the world and permission to be curious' (p.89). So the team must continually consider the linkage between different aspects of the child and her life so that unhelpful compartmentalization does not creep in.

The therapeutic parenting team, therapist and life-story worker each make a plan for their own area of work, based on their shared understanding of the child. Each plan is shared within the whole of the recovery team so everyone knows what is happening. The involvement of the whole recovery team in this way helps to ensure that there is a highly consistent and reliable approach to the child, running through the whole of her experience. This degree of safety, reliability and routine can play a very significant part in the recovery from trauma (*see* Chapter 3). It also enables unmet needs to be targeted in a focused way. The plans are discussed with the child so that she can agree ways forward and tailor the detail in her own way. For this purpose, child-friendly versions of the plan have been devised.

To illustrate how this works the following text is part of a therapeutic parenting plan for Grace, beginning with the first plan and then showing how the plan progressed over time.

Therapeutic parenting plan
BEDTIMES

- **Description:** This is an area where Grace exercises her need to be in control. She is often disruptive while others are being put to bed. She makes a lot of noise, shouting and banging her walls, and can become aggressive to adults. Grace usually enjoys a good bedtime with an adult, but can spoil it afterwards by disrupting others.

- **Understanding:** This may be down to Grace always wanting to be at the centre of everything, and needing to be involved in what is going on. She has also stated that she has sexual thoughts when in bed and thinks about one of the other children, Beth. When alone in her room her mind is very active and her head is full of things she doesn't want to think about. She may also feel unsafe at bedtime as this has been a time when she has experienced abuse and neglect.

- **Aims:** To enable Grace to feel safe and secure at bedtime and not need to control the situation. To allow her to settle to bed and feel relaxed. Enable her to express her fears and worries rather than internalizing them.

- **Plan:** To ensure boundaries around bedtime are consistent, but allow Grace to feel some control over her own routine, such as choosing her story and other things she likes to do.

Half an hour before bedtime, remind Grace that it will soon be bedtime. Make sure that her bed is made during the day and that her room feels cosy, for example, curtains drawn before dark. Help Grace to make her room a place she likes to be by putting nice things around her: pictures, books and toys. At bedtime encourage her to draw and colour, and to listen to soothing music as this helps her to relax. Give her the opportunity to talk about things which may be on her mind earlier in the evening, well before bedtime. To stay with her if she becomes disruptive and let her know that you will be with her and keep her safe no matter what she does. Make sure that Grace has had a wash and brushed her teeth before settling. She often likes her carer to be with her while she does this.

The important thing in the above plan is not so much some of the basic good care that is involved, but the way in which aspects of it are clearly related to an understanding of Grace and her history and, most of all, how everyone will be consistent in their approach.

THREE MONTHS LATER

This is an area of great improvement for Grace. There are very few disruptive bedtimes and she now chooses to sleep with her light and music off. She has recently shown greater need for reassurance and adult proximity, sometimes needing more time from adults. We think this is due to heightened anxieties following contact with mum and renewed thoughts of her foster mother's death.

SIX MONTHS LATER

Grace has a new bedtime routine and goes to bed at 9 pm. There is more time to sit and relax, and talk to an adult before bedtime. Use this time to sit with Grace, paying close attention to her mood and encourage her to talk.

EIGHT MONTHS LATER

Grace often uses the time before bed to try to take control. This may be by disrupting other children by being noisy, winding up others before their bedtime and trying to take control of the television. This may be due to heightened anxiety about her attachment to her key carer Susan. Since she has allowed Susan to 'look after her' she has become quite clingy and jealous of attention Susan gives to other children. Need to reflect empathetically to Grace what she is doing. Give her lots of reassurance that she doesn't need to do this. Grown-ups must all be consistent, stay in charge and manage this behaviour. Ensure that Grace's bedtime routine is reliable and, in particular, support Susan so that she is able to do this work.

ONE YEAR LATER

Bedtimes now mostly OK. Although in recent months, with some changes of adults and two children moving on, Grace has on occasions been very slow to settle even after good bedtimes, pottering about in her room until 11 pm or 12 am. Continue with original plan.

ONE YEAR AND EIGHT MONTHS LATER

Bedtimes largely good so Grace enjoys chatting to grown-ups during her bedtimes generally about fashion, room décor and things that have been happening during the day. She does not potter about until late anymore.

From this point onwards bedtimes ceased to be a problem for Grace and became a time of day that she enjoyed and was normally followed by a good night's sleep.

Relationships with staff and special provision

- **Description:** Grace resents being parented and tries to control all adults. She thinks she can look after herself and everybody else and does not need the grown-ups. She shows affection to the grown-ups but this is felt to be very superficial and can feel inappropriate. Grace finds it difficult to accept adult intervention and does not like being asked to do things. She shows little sign of real attachment. Grace arouses some feelings of dislike with some staff members, including her key carer.

- **Understanding:** Grace has had to look after herself and others, and does not believe that grown-ups can look after her and keep her safe. She has experienced people leaving her life, not being able to cope with her and even dying. Grown-ups cannot be relied upon. Grace's extreme dislike of herself may be transferred on to others. There has been a lack of positive males in her life.

- **Aims:** To enable Grace to form attachments and meaningful relationships. To facilitate her to allow herself to be parented and cared for. To help her to like herself. To help her form relationships with males.

- **Plan:** To give Grace lots of individual attention, in particular with her key carer, and introduce a male supporting carer to work alongside her key carer. To boost her self-esteem with plenty of praise, helping her to enjoy things she is good at and to support her in trying out new skills. To give lots of nurture and care, pre-empt her needs. To be aware that the way she makes us feel may reflect the way she feels. To empathize with her. To reflect the way she makes you feel by saying, for example, 'I'm feeling a bit uncomfortable at the moment, is that how you feel?' To show Grace that she can be cared for and nurtured despite these feelings. It is important that she does not feel that she overpowers her carers and that we are able to stay with her pain.

THREE MONTHS LATER

Grace shows signs of improvement in this area and is starting to attach to her key carer, Susan. As well as enjoying time with Susan, Grace is also testing her and pushes her away. Grace has recently allowed herself to behave as a little child when distressed, and responded very well to the nurture offered.

SIX MONTHS LATER

Grace's attachment with Susan continues to grow. Grace is also showing more trust of her supporting carer who is male (Tony). Susan and Tony to spend some joint time with Grace so that she can see they are working positively together. To continue to provide good experiences which Grace enjoys, such as cycling with Susan.

EIGHT MONTHS LATER

Grace is currently rejecting the adults to some degree, as she probably sees them as being unreliable (there had been staff absences owing to sickness and her therapist was also leaving). It is important to help Grace acknowledge her sense of loss and anger. To reassure her that she can still be cared for by giving lots of nurture. To support Susan with Grace's negativity, which Grace aims mostly at her.

ONE YEAR LATER

Grace's attachments seem more stable and she is at ease with various team members, including males. She says she likes Susan as her key carer except when she is angry with her, when she will say she wants a new one. Grace coped well when one of the team left and no longer struggles when someone comes back from annual leave or sickness.

ONE YEAR AND EIGHT MONTHS LATER

Grace is finding the lack of progress with family contact difficult and blames this on the house manager and Susan. When she is highly anxious she can revert to earlier attachment behaviour, such as pushing adults away or becoming overly dependent. Adults to remain positive about supporting Grace with her anxieties. She needs to see that the adults are going to care for her in the same way as before. Firm, consistent boundaries are needed. To help Grace to find ways of discussing her anxieties and praise her when she does this.

Through the rest of Grace's placement she continued to build attachments and largely use these relationships in a healthy way, though when faced with significant change or unsettling situations she would show some underlying insecurity. She made major progress in her capacity to form positive attachments, with both males and females, and to trust that these relationships would not harm her. However, due to her very difficult formative experiences Grace would need a highly supportive and understanding family environment to consolidate her growth. Grace did go on to make a positive transition to a family placement. The way in which she was able to separate from her key carer and home at Beech House and begin with her new family showed that she was now a far more resilient child.

Conclusion and further development

The SACCS' assessment process has now been running for over four years and has proved to be a useful treatment tool. A survey in 2006 involving 50 practitioners, found that 90 per cent agreed with the statement that 'the assessment and plan process helps children to achieve positive outcomes' and 98 per cent agreed that 'the assessment and plan process has enabled therapeutic parenting, life story and therapy practitioners to work more effectively together as a recovery team'.

However, fewer agreed that 'the assessment and plan process has enabled children to be more effectively involved in their own recovery'. This is an area that needs to be developed. SACCS is presently working on a format for children to evaluate their own progress, more clearly define their own outcomes and give feedback on the service provided. Potentially this could lead to the child's own picture of her progress being plotted on the spider diagram. This would provide another illuminating piece of information. For example, how would we consider a child whom practitioners considered to be well developed but the child's perception was much less positive? A consistency between the recovery team's view of the child and the child's own view could be an important factor in evaluating recovery. As well as adding the child's perspective, additional perspectives could also be gained from anyone else who might be closely involved, such as a teacher.

It is clear that the spider diagram is a useful and striking visualization of a child's progress. The same format could be adapted to show the progress of different user groups and for different outcomes. It can also be used for groups as well as individuals. For example, at SACCS the progress of different cohorts of children is being tracked using the average scores for each of the groups. This may give a clear picture of a group's overall progress and reveal differences between groups, to highlight, for instance, whether equality outcomes are being achieved between different gender, age and ethnic groups.

The assessment format clearly has a subjective element and further research is necessary to determine how reliably it provides an indicator of recovery, especially in the long term. It does, however, seem that the assessment and plan process helps to achieve many of the aspirations we have outlined in this book.

Notes

1. Easterbrook has given a detailed description of several methods of assessment and then considered their advantages and disadvantages. This chapter gratefully draws on her work on two of these assessments: Dockar-Drysdale's needs assessment and the Boxall Profile. For further information *see* Easterbrook (2006).

2. This model is described in detail in Kane (2007) and on which part of the chapter is based and gratefully acknowledged.

3. *See also* Bowlby (1969, 1973–1980), Howe (1995) and Howe *et al.* (1999).

4. The largest study was carried out by Susan Isaacs in the *Cambridge Evacuation Survey* (1941), which she edited. This covered all aspects of the evacuation, including physical condition. Work by Bannister and Ravden (1944) suggested that children might need psychological help. However, although stress was noted, it was found that the children who suffered psychological problems when evacuated tended to be those who had problems when at home.

5. For a concise explanation of how the brain develops, works and the impact which abuse and trauma can have on it *see* Pughe and Philpot (2007). For a summary of research *see* Glaser (2001) and Balbernie (2001).

6. Dysregulation of affect is when emotions seem out of control: the person feels that they are about to burst with emotion and overwhelm themselves and others with it if allowed to do so. For children, this can show itself in play by fantasy, movement, speaking almost in voices together with uncontrolled emotional outbursts unrelated to the play. Dysregulation of affect can show in children being defiant, anxious, unco-operative, depressed, impulse-ridden, acting unpredictably and being oppositional (James 1994).

7. The terms 'involvement', 'consultation', 'partnership', 'participation' and 'control', as applied to the part which users can play in the shaping and planning of services, are often used interchangeably. They may differ according to which group of service users is being discussed – as in the case here where reference is made to children and young people – but broad definitions are given in Philpot (1994).

References

Adcock, M. (2001) 'The core assessment process. How to synthesise information and make judgements.' In J. Horwath (ed.) *The Child's World. Assessing Children in Need.* London: Jessica Kingsley Publishers.

Aiyebusi, A. (2004) 'Touch and the impact of trauma in therapy relationships with adults.' In K. White (ed.) *Touch: Attachment and the Body.* London: Karnac Books.

Aldgate, J., Jones, D., Rose, W. and Jeffrey, C. (2006) *The Developing World of the Child.* London and Philadelphia: Jessica Kingsley Publishers.

Alvarez, A. (1992) *Live Company: Psychoanalytic Psychotherapy with Autistic, Borderline, Deprived and Abused Children.* London: Routledge.

Archer, C. (2003) 'Weft and warp: Developmental impact of trauma and implications for healing.' In C. Archer and A. Burnell (eds) *Trauma, Attachment and Permanence: Fear Can Stop You Loving.* London: Jessica Kingsley Publishers.

Balbernie, R. (2001) 'Circuits and circumstances: The neurobiological consequences of early relationship experiences and how they shape later behaviour.' *Journal of Child Psychotherapy 27*, 237–255.

Ball, S., Mudd, J., Nicholas, E., Oxley, M., Pinnock, M. and Qureshi, H. (2004) 'Make outcomes your big idea: Using outcomes to refocus social care practice and information.' *Journal of Integrated Care 12*, 5, 13–19.

Banks, N. (2001) 'Assessing children who belong to minority ethnic groups.' In J. Horwath (ed.) *The Child's World. Assessing Children in Need.* London: Jessica Kingsley Publishers.

Bannister, H. and Ravden, H. (1944) 'The problem child and his environment.' *British Journal of Psychology XXIV*, January.

Bennathan, M. and Boxall, M. (1998) *The Boxall Profile Handbook for Teachers.* London: Social and Emotional Difficulties Association.

Beresford, P. and Croft, S. (1980) *Community Control of Social Services Departments.* London: Battersea Community Action.

Bowlby, J. (1953) *Attachment and Loss, Volume 1.* London: Hogarth Press/Penguin.

Bowlby, J. (1969) *Attachment.* London: Hogarth Press.

Bowlby, J. (1973–1980) *Attachment Trilogy 1–111.* London: Hogarth Press.

Buckley, H. (2007) 'An integrated response to child neglect.' Address to 'Child Neglect: The Most Neglected Abuse' conference held by *Community Care*, 19 April.

Burnell, A. and Archer, C. (2003) 'Setting up the loom: Attachment theory revisited.' In C. Archer and A. Burnell (eds) *Trauma, Attachment and Permanence: Fear Can Stop You Loving.* London: Jessica Kingsley Publishers.

Cairns, K. (2002) *Attachment, Trauma and Resilience. Therapeutic Caring for Children.* London: British Association for Adoption and Fostering.

Cant, D. (2002) '"Joined-up psychotherapy": The place of individual psychotherapy in residential therapeutic provision for children.' *Journal of Child Psychotherapy 28,* 267–281.

Clifford-Poston, A. (2001) *The Secrets of Successful Parenting.* Oxford: How To Books.

Clough, R., Bullock, R. and Ward, A. (2006) *What Works in Residential Child Care. A Review of Research Evidence and the Practical Considerations.* London: National Children's Bureau.

Connor, T., Sclare, I., Dunbar, D. and Elliffe, J. (1985) 'Making a life story book.' *Adoption and Fostering 9,* 2.

Cox, A. and Bentovim, A. (2000) *Framework for the Assessment of Children in Need and Their Families. The Family Pack of Questionnaires and Scales.* London: The Stationery Office.

Crittenden, P.M. (1997) 'Toward an integrated theory of trauma.' In D. Cichetti and S.L. Tooth (eds) *The Rochester Symposium on Developmental Psychopathology.* New York, NY: University of Rochester Press.

Curtis, P. and Owen, P. (n.d.) 'Techniques of Working with Children.' Unpublished document.

Dalzell, R. and Sawyer, E. (2007) *Putting Analysis into Assessment: Undertaking Assessment of Need – A Toolkit for Practitioners.* London: National Children's Bureau Enterprises.

Department for Education and Employment (DfEE) (1997) *Excellence for all Children: Meeting Special Education Needs.* London: Department for Education and Skills.

Department of Health (DoH) (1989) *Caring for People: Community Care in the Next Decade and Beyond.* London: HMSO.

Department of Health (DoH) and Department for Education and Employment (DfEE) (2000) *Framework for Assessment of Children in Need and Their Families.* London: The Stationery Office.

Department of Health (DoH), Home Office and Department for Education and Employment (DfEE) (1999) *Working Together to Safeguard Children.* London: The Stationery Office.

Dockar-Drysdale, B. (1968) *Therapy in Child Care.* London: Longman.

Dockar-Drysdale, B. (1970) 'Need Assessment – 1, Finding a Basis, and Need Assessment – 11, Making an Assessment.' In B. Dockar-Drysdale (1993) *Therapy and Consultation in Child Care.* London: Free Association Books.

Dockar-Drysdale, B. (1973) *Consultation in Child Care.* London: Longman.

Dockar-Drysdale, B. (1990) *The Provision of Primary Experience.* London: Free Association Books.

Dockar-Drysdale, B. (1993) *Therapy and Consultation in Child Care.* London: Free Association Books.

Easterbrook, L. (2006) 'Does the SACCS' Assessment Process Contribute to the "Recovery" of Traumatized Children in the Area of Attachment?' Unpublished MA thesis.

Fahlberg, V. (1994) *A Child's Journey Through Placement.* London: British Association for Adoption and Fostering.

Flynn, D. (1998) 'In-patient work in a therapeutic community.' In M. Lanyado and A. Horne (eds) *The Handbook of Child and Adolescent Psychotherapy: Psychoanalytic Approaches.* London: Routledge.

Gibson, F. (2004) *The Past in the Present. Reminiscence Work in Health and Social Care.* Baltimore, MD: Health Professions Press.

Glaser, D. (2001) 'Child abuse, neglect and the brain: A review.' *Journal of Child Psychology and Psychiatry and Allied Disciplines 41*, 97–116.

Haight, B. (1998) 'Use of life review/life story books in families with Alzheimer's disease.' In P. Schweitzer (ed.) *Reminiscence in Dementia Care.* London: Age Exchange.

Hart, B. and Risley, T.R. (2002) *Meaningful Differences in the Everyday Experience of Young American Children.* Baltimore, MD: Paul Brookes Publishing Co.

Harvey, J. (2006) *Valuing and Educating Young People: Stern Love the Lyward Way.* London and Philadelphia: Jessica Kingsley Publishers.

HM Treasury (2003) *Every Child Matters.* London: The Stationery Office.

Horwath, J. (2001) 'Assessing the world of the child in need. Background and context.' In J. Horwath, (ed.) *The Child's World. Assessing Children in Need.* London: Jessica Kingsley Publishers.

House of Commons (1998) *Second Report of the Health Select Committee – Children Looked After by Local Authorities* (HC 319-1). London: The Stationery Office.

Howe, D. (1995) *Attachment Theory for Social Work Practice.* Basingstoke: Macmillan.

Howe, D. (2000) 'Attachment.' In M. Davies (ed.) *The Blackwell Encyclopaedia of Social Work.* Oxford: Blackwell.

Howe, D., Brandon, M., Hinings, D. and Schofield, G. (1999) *Attachment Theory, Child Maltreatment and Family Support.* Basingstoke: Macmillan.

Hunter, M. (2001) *Psychotherapy and Young People in Care: Lost and Found.* Hove: Brunner-Routledge.

Isaacs, S. (1941) (ed.) *Cambridge Evacuation Survey.* London: Methuen.

James, B. (1994) *Handbook for Treatment of Attachment-Trauma Problems in Children.* New York, NY: Free Press.

Jordan, B. (2007) *Social Work and Well-Being.* Lyme Regis: Russell House Publishing.

Kane, S. (2007) *Care Planning for Children in Residential Care.* London: National Children's Bureau.

Kelly, J.G. (1974) 'Toward a psychology of healthiness.' Ichabod Spencer Lecture, Union College, Schenectady, NY.

Kennell, J., Voos, D. and Klaus, M. (1976); cited in V. Fahlberg (1979) *Attachment and Separation.* Michigan: Department of Social Services; cited in L. Easterbrook (2006) *Does the SACCS Assessment Process Contribute to the 'Recovery' of Traumatized Children in the Area of Attachment?* University of Reading: Unpublished MA thesis.

Laming, Lord (2003) *Inquiry into the Death of Victoria Climbié.* London: The Stationery Office.

Layard, R. (2005) *Happiness: Lessons from a New Science.* London: Penguin Books.

Levy, T.M. and Orlans, M. (1998) *Attachment, Trauma and Healing: Understanding and Treating Attachment Disorder in Children and Families.* Washington, DC: CWLA Press.

Lyward, G. (1958) *Unlabelled Living.* Conference talk for the Residential Care of Disturbed Children, National Association for Mental Health, 5–11 March.

Mabey, R. (2005) *Nature Cure.* London: Chatto & Windus.

Menzies-Lyth, I. (1988) *Containing anxiety in institutions: Selected Essays Vol 1.* London: Free Association Books.

Milner, J. and O'Byrne, P. (2002) *Assessment in Social Work.* Basingstoke: Palgrave Macmillan.

Parry, G. and Richardson, A. (1996) *NHS Psychotherapy Services in England: Review of Strategic Policy.* London: NHS Executive.

Perry, B. (1999) 'The memories of states: How the brain receives and retrieves traumatic experience.' In J. Goodwin and R. Attias (eds) *Splintered Reflections. Images of the Body in Trauma.* New York, NY: Basic Books.

Perry, B. and Szalavitz, M. (2006) *The Boy Who Was Raised as a Dog.* New York, NY: Basic Books.

Philpot, T. (1994) *Managing to Listen. A Guide to User Involvement for Mental Health Service Managers.* London: King's Fund.

Pithers, W.D., Gray, A., Busconi, A. and Houchhenns, P. (1998) 'Children with sexual behaviour problems: Identification of five distinct types and related treatment considerations.' *Child Maltreatment 5,* 4, 384–406.

Pointon, C. (2004) 'The future of trauma work.' *CPJ on line.* Accessed on 16/10/07 at www.bacp.co.uk/cpj/may2004/trauma.htm

Prickett, J. (1974) 'A memorial address.' *New Era 55,* 3, 53–59.

Prior, V. and Glaser, D. (2006) *Understanding Attachment and Attachment Disorders.* London and Philadelphia: Jessica Kingsley Publishers.

Pughe, B. and Philpot, T. (2007) *Living Alongside a Child's Recovery: Therapeutic Parenting with Traumatized Children.* London and Philadelphia: Jessica Kingsley Publishers.

Raynes, B. (2006) 'Common ground?' *Community Care,* 9–15 February.

Rilke, H. (1903) 'Letter to Frank Xaver Kappus' (translated by Jennifer Cole). Quoted in J. Harvey (2006) *Valuing and Educating Young People: Stern Love the Lyward Way.* London and Philadelphia: Jessica Kingsley Publishers.

Rose, R. and Philpot, T. (2005) *The Child's Own Story: Life Story Work with Traumatized Children.* London: Jessica Kingsley Publishers.

Rowe, J. (1980) 'Fostering in the 1970s and beyond.' In J. Triseliotis (ed.) *New Developments in Foster Care and Adoption.* London: Routledge.

Ryan, T. and Walker, R. (2003) *Life Story Work: A Practical Guide to Helping Children Understand Their Past.* London: British Association for Adoption and Fostering.

Rymaszewska, J. and Philpot, T. (2006) *Reaching the Vulnerable Child: Therapy with Traumatized Children.* London and Philadelphia: Jessica Kingsley Publishers.

Sawyer, L. (2005) 'An outcome-based approach to domiciliary care.' *Journal of Integrated Care 13,* 3, 20–25.

Schore, A.N. (1994) *Affect Regulation and the Origin of the Self: The Neurobiology of Emotional Development.* New Jersey: Erlbaum.

Sinclair, R. (1991) *Residential Care and the Children Act 1989.* London: National Children's Bureau.

Sinclair, R., Garrett, L. and Berridge, D. (1995) *Social Work and Assessment with Adolescents.* London: National Children's Bureau.

Social Services Inspectorate (1991) *Care Management and Assessment: A Managers' Guide.* London: HMSO.

Solomon, J. and George, C.C. (eds) (1999) *Attachment Disorganization.* New York, NY: Guildhall Press.

Stevenson, O. (1998) *Neglected Children: Issue and Dilemmas.* Oxford: Blackwell.

Timms, J.E. and Thoburn, J. (2003) *Your Shout! A Survey of the Views of 706 Children and Young People in Public Care.* London: NSPCC.

Tomlinson, P. (in press), 'Assessing the needs of traumatized children to improve outcomes.' *Journal of Social Work Practice.*

Thompson, N. (2000) *Theory and Practice in Human Services.* Maidenhead: Open University Press.

Toynbee, P. (2004) 'We can break the vice of the great unmentionable.' *Guardian*, 2 January.

van der Kolk, B. (2002) 'In terror's grip: Healing the ravages of trauma.' *Cerebrum 4*, 34–50.

van der Kolk, B., McFarlane, A.C. and Weisaeth, L. (1996) *Traumatic Stress: The Effects of Overwhelming Experience on Mind, Body and Society*. New York, NY: Guilford Publications.

Vygotsky, L.S. (1978) *Mind and Society. The Development of Higher Mental Processes*. Cambridge, MA: Harvard University Press.

Walsh, M. (2002) '24 outcomes for recovery.' In M. Walsh and P. Tomlinson (eds), *The SACCS' Recovery Programme*. Unpublished text.

Ward, A. (2004) 'Assessing and meeting children's emotional needs.' Lecture notes for address at the therapeutic child care study day, University of Reading organized by the University of Reading.

Ward, H. (1996) 'Constructing and implementing measures to assess the outcomes of looking after children away from home.' In M. Hill and J. Aldgate (eds) *Child Welfare Services: Developments in Law, Policy, Practice and Research*. London: Jessica Kingsley Publishers.

Williams, A. and McCann, J. (2006) *Care Planning for Looked After Children: A Toolkit for Practitioners*. London: National Children's Bureau.

Willis, M. (2001) 'Outcomes in social care: Conceptual confusion and practical impossibility?' In *Leadership for Social Care Outcomes Module Handbook 2005*. Institute of Local Government Studies, University of Birmingham.

Winnicott, D.W. (1962) 'Ego integration in child development.' Republished in D.W. Winnicott (1990) *The Maturational Process and the Facilitating Environment*. London and New York: Karnac Books.

Winnicott, D. (1947) 'Hate in the counter transference.' In D. Winnicott (2002) *Through Paediatrics to Psychoanalysis*. London: Karnac Books.

Woods, J. (2003) *Boys Who Have Abused: Psychoanalytic Psychotherapy with Victim/Perpetrators of Sexual Abuse*. London and Philadelphia: Jessica Kingsley Publishers.

YoungMinds (2004) *Mental Health in Infancy*. London: YoungMinds.

Ziegler, D. (2002) *Traumatic Experience and the Brain. A Handbook for Understanding and Treating Those Traumatized as Children*. Phoenix, AZ: Acacia Publishing.

The Story of SACCS

In the 1960s and 1970s professionals focused on the physical abuse (or what was called the battered baby syndrome) and neglect of children. Sexual abuse only began to gain attention in the early 1980s.

The challenge then for social workers in child protection was to deal with this new phenomenon as part of everyday practice. They had to develop new skills to communicate with children on a subject which they, as adults, had difficulty with, that is talking about sex and their own sexuality, and moreover doing this in a way that could withstand in court the rigours of legal scrutiny.

It was at this point that Mary Walsh, now chief executive of SACCS, got together with a local authority colleague, Madge Bray, who was working to help disturbed children communicate by using toys. Together they looked at how they could adapt the use of the toy box to help this very vulnerable group of children communicate their distress, especially about the abuse they had suffered. Above all, they wanted to give children a voice in decisions which would be made about them, particularly in court.

SACCS comes into being

Working within the culture of uncertainty and confusion that prevailed at the time, Mary Walsh and Madge Bray became disenchanted at the lack of time and resources available to do this work properly. They saw no alternative: in January 1987 they took it upon themselves to meet the profound needs of the deeply traumatized children whom they were seeing every day and who found themselves effectively lost and without any influence on their futures.

SACCS came into being in Madge Bray's back bedroom – the typewriter had to be unplugged to use the photocopier! Demand for the venture on which they were now embarked soon became apparent. They were inundated with requests to see children and help them to communicate about their distress. Mary Walsh and Madge Bray worked with children all over the country, helping them to tell their stories, giving comfort and allowing them to express their pain. They also acted as advocates for children in court and other decision-making bodies, and as case consultants to local authorities. Through this process, as expected, they began to notice that many of the children were changing and beginning to find some resolution to their difficulties.

They also became aware that there were some very small children who, because of what had happened to them, were either too eroticized or too disturbed to be placed in foster care. Many foster carers who were not prepared or trained to deal with very challenging situations day to day would quickly become weighed down by the child's sexualized behaviour and the placement would break down. The real cause of these breakdowns was never acknowledged and therefore never dealt with. In time these children were labelled as unfosterable and placed in residential care along with much older children and young people.

Leaps and Bounds

The heartbreak of watching this happen to three-, four- and five-year-old children was unacceptable. The need was to be able to hold the children and their behaviour lovingly while they were helped to understand and deal with the root cause of their behaviour. The result was the setting up of Leaps and Bounds, the first SACCS residential care provision.

The birth was a long and difficult one, but after three years the first house, Hopscotch, was opened. It filled up immediately, and the children were cared for by staff trained to understand the issues and encouraged to put love into everything they did. Many of the children placed in Leaps and Bounds had experienced many placement break-downs. Some had been placed for adoption that had subsequently failed. Most had incoherent life histories. Some had lost touch with members of their family and one child, incredibly, had acquired the wrong name. The great need was to find all of this information that was lost in the system, and so the life-story service came into existence, to help to piece together the fabric of the children's lives and give them back their own identity.

In addition, a team of professional play therapists was engaged to work with the children in Hopscotch, and subsequently at the new houses – Somersault, Cartwheel, Handstand, Leapfrog and others – while continuing to bring the special SACCS approach to children who were not in residential care.

Within SACCS, all those charged with responsibility for the well-being of the child were (and are) expected to share information with each other, so that the whole team holds the child's reality and care.

Find Us, Keep Us

The expectation at SACCS was that when children had come to terms with what had happened to them and were ready to move on, their local authorities would find foster families for them. This proved not to be the case in many instances, and children who had worked hard to recover and desperately wanted to be part of a family would have their hopes dashed. As a result their behaviour deteriorated. It was extremely difficult to watch this happening, especially as the next part of the work needed to be done within a family.

Leaps and Bounds was never intended to become a permanent placement for the children, so looking for potential foster families and training them to care for this very challenging and vulnerable group of children became the responsibility of a new part of SACCS which was founded – Find Us, Keep Us, the fostering and family placement arm of the organization. Find Us, Keep Us became SACCS Family Placement in 2005.

Flying Colours

In 1997 Flying Colours was opened. It was a new project designed to meet the needs of young adolescents. Often these were children who had been traumatized when they were very young, but had only just started to talk about it. As a therapist, Mary Walsh had worked with many such young people, who were not being held in a safe and contained environment. She knew that they often ran away when feelings overwhelmed them, and sometimes ended up living hand to mouth on inner city streets, involved in prostitution, drug taking and worse. Flying Colours offered these young people the same loving and nurturing therapeutic care as the younger children in Leaps and Bounds whilst meeting their different developmental needs.

SACCS Care

In 2003, a major rationalization was undertaken to integrate all of the SACCS services which had evolved since the organization's early days. A new company, SACCS Care, was formed, with an organizational focus on the parenting aspect of therapeutic care. This is arguably the most important job carried out with children, some of whom have similar developmental profiles to the most dangerous adults in our society. SACCS believes that unless this issue is addressed properly, traumatized children cannot have a positive experience of parenting, and when the time comes will be unable to parent their own children appropriately.

The SACCS Recovery Programme

In 2006 SACCS launched an outcomes-based approach to the treatment of traumatized children, based on the unique SACCS 24 outcomes for recovery. This programme is supported by the assessment and planning process described in this book and has achieved national recognition as an example of excellent practice (Kane 2007).

Today and tomorrow

SACCS Care is differentiated by a unique integrated model of thera-peutic parenting, play therapy, life-story work and education support individually tailored to meet children's needs, coupled with a fostering service for those who are ready to move to a family.

At the time of writing, SACCS Care is a growing Midlands-based organization looking after 70 children and employing 175 profes-sional care staff and managers. The SACCS model is underpinned by a complex structure of practice training and clinical supervision, and these standards of excellence have positioned the organization as a national leader in therapeutic care and recovery.

There are many children outside SACCS struggling with the enormous trauma caused by abuse and neglect, children whose experi-ence has taught them that families are dangerous places in which to live. SACCS believes that every child has a right to the expert thera-peutic care which can help them to recover from their emotional injuries, but for these children the specialist services they require are often not available.

The Mary Walsh Institute

By 2006 SACCS had fully evolved to offer outstanding services for children, and at this pivotal point in the company's development its practitioners found themselves increasingly called upon to lecture to, and train, fellow professionals, both nationally and internationally. Again, the time was right for SACCS to develop a new service: the Mary Walsh Institute dedicated to improving outcomes and influenc-ing practice with traumatized children.

The institute will offer SACCS practice through a programme of higher education, vocational training, publications, research and con-sultancy. It now provides the foundation degree in therapeutic child care, provided by SACCS and the North East Wales Institute, part of the University of Wales, for the company's entire frontline workforce. This training ensures that all those engaged in direct work with children are fully trained and professionally equipped to carry out the roles which are central to recovery. From September 2007 an MA degree in Therapeutic Child Care will be offered in partnership with Liverpool Hope University and a BA degree is in development. The Mary Walsh Institute was launched in 2007 at the SACCS international conference on childhood trauma and recovery.

The Authors

Patrick Tomlinson is strategic development director and a member of the SACCS board. He has over 22 years' experience in work with traumatized children, as a practitioner, service manager and director. He began his career at the Cotswold Community, a therapeutic community for emotionally damaged boys. He spent 14 years there, the last six as Assistant Principal. Following a two-year period working with Young Options as Head of Therapy and Regional Director, he joined SACCS in 2002. His qualifications include an MA in therapeutic child care and Postgraduate Certificate in Strategic Social Care Leadership. He is the author of a number of papers and *Therapeutic Approaches in Work with Traumatised Children and Young People* (2004). Working with Mary Walsh, he has been central to the development of the SACCS Recovery Programme.

Terry Philpot is a journalist and writer and is a contributor to various publications. He has written and edited more than a dozen books, the latest of which are (with Anthony Douglas) *Adoption: Changing Families, Changing Times* (2002), (with Julia Feast) *Searching Questions. Identity, Origins and Adoption* (2003), (with Clive Sellick and June Thoburn) *What Works in Foster Care and Adoption?* (2004) and (with Richard Rose) *The Child's Own Story. Life Story Work with Traumatized Children* (2004), (with Janie Rymaszewska) *Reaching the Vulnerable Child. Therapy with Traumatized Children* (2006) and (with Billy Pughe) *Living Alongside a Child's Recovery. Therapeutic Parenting with Traumatized Children* (2007). He is currently writing a book on the partners of sex offenders. He has also published reports on private fostering and kinship care. His second report on residential care for older people run by the Catholic Church, *The Length of Days: How Can the Church Meet the Challenges of an Ageing Society?*, was published in 2007. He is a trustee of the Michael Sieff Foundation and the Social Care Institute for Excellence and was formerly a trustee of Rainer. He has won several awards for journalism.

Subject Index

Author Index